Praise for *This Won't Hurt*

'Marieke is balanced in her evidence analysis,
forensic in her research' *Telegraph*

'A hugely informative and quietly furious call
to arms . . . with the skill and methodological
precision of a surgeon' *Irish Times*

'A ground-breaking new book' *Evening Standard*

'Asking all the right questions about the treatment
of women's bodies and more importantly, answering
them. Punchy, fascinating and vital' *Rachel Parris*

'A vital subject that needs to be discussed' *Katy Hessel*

'A valuable sociological perspective on women's bodies
and health and an even more valuable (and optimistic)
view of a better future for all' *Gina Rippon*

'A brilliant book . . . There is so much to unlearn,
there is so much that also follows in terms of how
medicine could support – rather than fail – half
the world's population' *Helen Pankhurst*

T0371893

Dr Marieke Bigg holds a PhD in sociology from the University of Cambridge. Her work focused on the role of biological models and biologists in public deliberations on biotechnology and reproductive medicine. She also writes fiction that deals with the intersection of art and the female body. Besides her writing, she runs writing workshops, lectures, and collaborates with scientists and artists to produce exhibitions that conjure new social worlds.

This Won't Hurt

How Medicine Fails Women

Dr Marieke Bigg

HODDER &
STOUGHTON

First published in Great Britain in 2023 by Hodder & Stoughton Limited
An Hachette UK company

The authorised representative in the EEA is Hachette Ireland, 8 Castlecourt
Centre, Dublin 15, D15 XTP3, Ireland (email: info@hbgi.ie)

This paperback edition published in 2024

5

Image Permissions: p.5 © Shubhangi Ganeshrao Kene/Getty Images/Science Photo
Library RF; p.27 Used with permission from the Better for Women 2019 report, RCOG
© the Royal College of Obstetricians & Gynaecologists; p.68 Creative Commons, from
the Mauritshuis Online Catalogue; p.176 from C H Waddington, *Organisers and Genes*
frontispiece, 1940; p.176 from C H Waddington, *Strategies of the Genes*; p.241 Creative
Commons, from Marie Docher/Odile Fillod; p.252 Courtesy of the Laboratory for Tissue
Engineering and Organ Fabrication, Massachusetts General Hospital, Boston, MA, USA,
Dr Joseph Vacanti; p.259 Concept and Design: Hendrik-Jan Grievink (Next Nature)/
Photography: Digidaan; p.273 used with permission from the artist, Suzanne Anker.

A CIP catalogue record for this title is available from the British Library

Paperback ISBN 978 1 529 37772 9
ebook ISBN 978 1 529 37770 5

Typeset in Bembo MT by Hewer Text UK Ltd, Edinburgh
Printed and bound in Great Britain by Clays Ltd, Elcograf S.p.A.

Hodder & Stoughton policy is to use papers that are natural, renewable
and recyclable products and made from wood grown in sustainable forests.
The logging and manufacturing processes are expected to conform
to the environmental regulations of the country of origin.

Hodder & Stoughton Limited
Carmelite House
50 Victoria Embankment
London EC4Y 0DZ

www.hodder.co.uk

Contents

Part 3 – Future Bodies

To all those humans who want enough for their bodies, so that they can be more than their bodies.

A note on terminology

This book points to the vast unexplored territory that has, so far, remained beyond the purview of patriarchal science. In order to show how science has formed around the interests of bodies that fell into the category of 'man', I discuss how it has excluded the bodies that fall into the category of 'woman'. I made the choice to do so in order to gesture to science's blind-spots using a language that we know and share; I use the terms 'man' and 'woman' strategically, but they are far from definitive, and they are certainly not an end-point.

Throughout this book, I use the term 'woman' to show how scientists have looked for biological evidence to reinforce their socially constructed idea of what a woman is. I use the term woman to connote the historical, gendered connotations that came to be associated with that cluster of biological traits and that have been used to oppress and exclude these othered bodies from medicine and society – be it weakness, irregularity, or degeneracy, or the social roles of childbearer and mother. The category of woman was built using biological traits.

Illuminating the exclusion of women is only the beginning. I want to show how new research is pushing the boundaries of the neat and tidy categories of man and woman we thought we knew: the real experiences of women in their bodies that challenge the social roles ascribed to them; the real findings in science that complicate the biological picture of a woman as a body with a specific anatomy, and hormones, and behaviour. The experiences of women with aspects of 'male' anatomy, and vice versa, that are leading scientists to re-evaluate their understanding of biologically rooted assumptions about both sex and gender.

The assumptions we hold about gender were never written into biology, but were constructed, through time, in a social context, by scientists *using* biology. Some of the most exciting new avenues of research that can help us break with old biological gendered categories are being conducted by scientists, often women, taking up biology in new ways to answer the questions that matter to people who don't fall into the historical and biological category of 'man'. This is exciting and relevant research to those who identify as women, as it comes with the added benefit of a better understanding of how biology actually works. Throughout this book, I make the case that science that moves beyond the restrictive purview of gendered categories is also a better science. It is exciting to me that breaking with gendered ideas is synonymous with improving science. As we show that biology and social ideas don't align in the way that we thought, we grow a new repository of knowledge that can be used to grow understanding and claim legitimacy for the experiences of not only women but also intersex people, trans and nonbinary people, and with it, hopefully, find more adequate terminology. All this, while improving our understanding, scientifically, of how the human body works.

In this book, I hope to break open the categories of man and woman and let in some light. This is a starting point, it is stunted. I call for new language, but sometimes I revert to the restrictive language we hold. I call for a better representation of women in science, but sometimes the gender of the experts I consult reflects the state of a field still dominated by men. I call for greater attention to diverse patient voices, but beyond my personal experience, this book is comprised largely of the voices of scientists, academics and medical professionals. Nonetheless, this book is a tool, that I hope will be taken up by those whose bodies have existed in medical silence, to validate their experience, and to begin to draw shapes around new clusters of symptoms and experiences, to forge a path into that medical unknown.

This book is an invitation to all those patients, scientists and people who deserve better, and for whom science could do better, to tell their stories, in the words that they can find, until we find new ones, that come closer to the truth.

Introduction: A 'Natural' Woman

I visited the gynaecologist recently to try to get to the bottom of a chronic problem – a mysterious feeling in my nether-regions I could only describe vaguely as 'discomfort' or 'pressure'. I had no words for it, no medical verb like 'itching' or 'burning' or 'throbbing', and so the gynaecologist didn't really know what to do with me. He sent me for an ultrasound. Laying there with my legs hoisted up, and a dildo-like device pushed inside of me, I experienced a moment of extreme emptiness. I associated ultrasounds with pregnancy – a doctor pointing to a blip on the screen, a couple gazing lovingly at their pea-sized prospect of a person. I wasn't shown the image of whatever they were trying to locate inside of me. I knew it wasn't a baby. But that wasn't the problem. The particular emptiness I felt didn't come from the absence of life. It came from the gaping void in my vocabulary. It came from my sense of utter disconnection from the process unfolding at the other end of the inspection table. It came from not knowing what was wrong with me. From not even knowing what my doctor was looking for.

When I met my gynaecologist for the much-anticipated follow-up appointment, he could tell me very little. No cysts, he said, no tumours – nothing lethal. Might be endometriosis, he suggested, and casually offered me the option of keyhole surgery to further investigate the cause. This would involve an anaesthetic, after which they would cut into my belly and insert a camera to inspect the inside of my womb. I'd come to the appointment expecting scientific images of my uterus; instead, I was left with one of my body as an inanimate object, a keyhole waiting for the insertion of a pretty noncommittal medical key. I politely declined. The gynaecologist nodded and said it wasn't a problem. I wondered how it possibly could have been a problem, whom it could have posed a problem for. He added: 'Maybe next time I see you, it'll be for a happy occasion. Maybe in the maternity unit.'

I was left wondering if I looked like I was approaching the end of my childbearing window. In one way, that was insulting: I was twenty-eight and surely had a few years to go. In another way though, those words, coming from a man in a white coat, a man so learned and established, in a setting so clinical and authoritative, were exciting, *thrilling*. Thrilling in the sense that I could be considered that uncomplicated idea of a woman – just a body waiting to conceive. You see, I've never been able to view my body with the kind of assurance that this doctor was doing.

I've spent my whole life wanting to be a 'natural' woman. And by that, I mean I've always wanted to *feel* the things I thought other girls felt, to pass the milestones other female bodies went through. I assumed this journey was effortless for other women; it appeared to be from the outside. Then again, from the outside, I must have also presented like an effortless girl. I look like your most generic of cis females: boobs, curves, silky hair and bright clothes to match. Inside, though, I've always felt like an imposter. Mainly because I have always felt as though my body was betraying me.

When I tried inserting a tampon for the first time, it wasn't smooth and empowering like it seemed to be for the other girls at school – I panicked and fainted at the thought that it might get stuck.

When I had sex for the first time, it wasn't like a whole new world had opened up – it hurt, and I was scared that we'd done some irreparable damage.

When I started taking the contraceptive pill, it wasn't this cool little moment where the alarm on your phone went off and you popped one like a tab of LSD in front of your friends and got on with your life – my boobs swelled to three times their normal size and, emotionally, I felt like the end was nigh.

At every biological juncture in my life, things haven't gone the way I've been taught they were supposed to, and so I've felt like a traitor to my sex. And right at the epicentre of my anxieties was the doctor's consultation room. I've always been anxious that medicine would expose me. Worried they'd find something: a deviancy or a deficiency in me. Abnormal periods, an unreceptive uterus – conclusive evidence that I am not a *proper* female.

I now know that many women have also experienced that discrepancy between inside and outside that I have often felt. I now know that we women spend our lives receiving strong messages about our bodies, about what is 'normal' or 'expected', and that those messages are often slippery and subversive, as they seep into our very being, guiding how we behave, what we choose to say and what we choose to keep to ourselves.

It's sometimes been hard to figure out who or what has been making me feel this way. The other girls at school, flaunting their tampons as if they were status symbols? TV telling me that I was going to orgasm from awkward missionary sex in under two seconds? Online culture, perhaps, with its celebration of a rendition of womanhood that has always seemed so clean, sexualised and unattainable? Or medicine? The doctors' comments, prescriptions and procedures that have all taken for granted what a 'normal' woman should be.

Now I accept that it's all of these things, and more – all of them entwined, reinforcing each other, conspiring to build an image of the female body so far removed from any individual actual female body. But where does that all begin? Where does it start?

From my own experience, I know that I picked up messages about my body gradually, iteratively. I was lucky enough – and many people aren't – to receive sex education at school, and the overall aura of hilarity and over-emphasis on genitals were something that definitely coloured my idea of the differences between boys and girls. But none of that was new. We'd all encountered 'pee-pees' before, and we'd already had the important discussion about which of the many holes between a girl's legs was for weeing and which for baby-making, an activity which, again, luckily for me, was totally mythical at the age of 10. All of this was vaguely entertaining, its meaning still in the making, but nonetheless very much present. The education I received in class was just the finesse, pre-empted and followed by a lifetime of subliminal messaging.

I remember how when I was about ten, my brother and I were fighting and he punched me in my lower abdomen. My grandma, who was walking us home from school, told him off, stating that he'd hit me in 'a very special area for girls'. I think that was the first time I became aware of my childbearing capacity. The first time I had a sense *that* thing, rather than my tenacity or creativity (the things my mum tended to emphasise), was what made me special.

I was a lucky child, in many ways. I was able to live and breathe and explore who I was for a long time before these constricting messages about being a baby-maker, about my body defining my value (and yet, at the same time, my body never being properly valued), began to filter through. Nonetheless, I wasn't impervious and, slowly, I was forced to grow up, to face the ideas and internalise the messages that define a woman through her body.

Challenging bikini biology

The idea that a woman is defined by her childbearing capacity is pervasive in our world. This is as true of medicine as it is of culture at large, but given the subtle and entangled ways in which people learn about these ideas, repeat them and internalise them until they feel so true they can only be *natural*, it can be hard to expose the sexist assumptions that travel between culture and medicine.

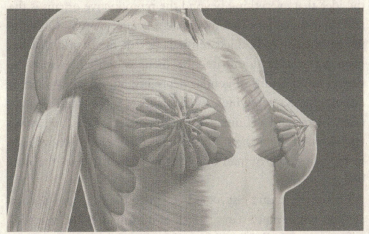

This image shows the musculature of a female body. The floral-shaped structures around the breasts are milk ducts.[1]

There are, however, moments when the relationship between sexist culture and the culture of medicine comes glaringly into view. In 2019, this image of the female musculature went viral (see page 5). But this wasn't the body we thought we knew. Thousands of Twitter users were amazed by the floral shape of the milk ducts, which, in contrast, were absent from the textbook images of the skeletal, nervous or muscular systems they'd come across in their school biology lessons. Those images rarely had breasts, usually sporting the square shoulders more typical to male musculature. And when female anatomy was ever discussed and some reference to a particular part of her anatomy was unavoidable, perhaps an image of the same male, 'normal' body was presented, only with a female reproductive system in situ.

This is because most of us would have been taught what Bart Fauser, University of Utrecht's Professor of Reproductive Medicine and Gynaecology, calls the 'bikini vision' of biology: the idea that everything beyond the reproductive organs is the same across genders; that medicine is gender neutral. Only the image of these milk ducts reminds us that in a world that has been historically dominated by men, we should always be suspicious of claims of gender neutrality, all too easily used to disguise the ways in which a male standard is upheld as normal, often better and definitely more important. Thus, when we take stock of the images used to reflect the state of knowledge in medicine, the human body seems really to mean the *male* body.

Of course, it isn't just regarding gynaecology where women are met with empty stares, a lack of information and inappropriate care. The bikini vision of biology blinds and misleads researchers across all fields of medicine, blocks avenues to funding based on a general reluctance to invest in female-specific questions and misdirects doctors in their diagnosis and treatment of patients.

The female body works differently from the male, and not only in terms of reproductive abilities – from hearts to hormones to genes, we differ down to our very cells. This means that we also face different risk factors when it comes to specific diseases and that they may arise at different moments in our lives and in a sex-specific way. Yet medicine isn't equipped to take heed of these differences. And, for the vast majority of human history, medicine didn't even notice these differences.

Take heart disease for example: a leading cause of death worldwide across genders, but still often considered a male disease. A large group of symptoms long discarded as atypical in cardiology is slowly being recognised as specific to the female manifestation of the disease. Most women don't feel that classic chest pain we see in TV dramas – instead, fatigue, nausea, jaw, back or arm pain or shortness of breath are more common. In the case of transgender men and women, research into how heart attack symptoms present is even more limited. Because these symptoms deviate from the male model of the disease, heart disease in women and othered bodies has often been left undiagnosed, and so untreated. Women are still less likely to undergo heart test checks such as coronary angiography (an X-ray for the coronary arteries), to receive treatment like stents or heart surgery or take medication. How can we get the help we need when studies show that those women who have had a heart attack are 59% more likely than men to receive the wrong diagnosis from the start? You can't treat a disease when the diagnosis is wrong.

When the male default is overall still considered to be neutral, visions of a specifically female biology and entirely different bodies are almost inconceivable – and that is what **Part 1** of this book deals with, addressing those areas of research that have been neglected as a result of this preoccupation with male biology. There is a whole complex system that has been relegated to the shadows because the male anatomy has been the default. This has also meant that women's pain and symptoms have often been disregarded and/or ignored.

In **Part 2, Misconceived Bodies**, we see how female bodies have not only been ignored but also misunderstood, in part as a result of the assumption that the male body was the default, but also due to gendered ideas about femaleness and women. This misconception is what led doctors to discard female-specific symptoms for heart disease as atypical, while drugs and treatment, such as the classic defibrillation, were developed for what was considered a predominantly 'male' disease. It is also what has led doctors to treat male and female bodies with the same pain medication, when females embody entirely different pain signalling pathways requiring different interventions.

Part 3, Future Bodies, asks how we can look to the new futuristic possibilities emerging in medicine to ensure that we serve the needs of all bodies. From femtech to artificial wombs, this section offers science fictions on the verge of becoming realities and shows how the ideas about gender shaping their design and implementation will determine whether we progress onto utopian or dystopian futures.

I am a cisgender woman and that is the story that I, from my position in this world, feel most capable of telling, so the focus of this book is inadvertently on cisgender women. In its course, I touch on how the medical neglect of cisgender women is entwined with the medical neglect of people of colour, transgender people and intersex people and anyone who doesn't fit the default white, male (and heterosexual) focus of modern medicine. There are so many more stories to be told than I can tell, and I want to acknowledge that from the outset.

There is also, I admit, comparatively more research on cis-female bodies than on transgender women or on women of colour – in medicine, these are groups of people relegated to an even more distant beyond. Yet I hope that this story provides some recognition and information for people in all of these other bodies, and that at the very least, I can know some of my unknowns, and point to directions in which others might venture.

Some of my story will be relevant to some of the other 'others' in medicine, and for this reason 'woman' can be read as shorthand for 'women and differently gendered', because these bodies all fall out of the purview of mainstream medicine. I will not pretend that the information I provide is attuned to the specificities of the experiences of the groups to which I don't belong, but I do believe that for most whose medical problems form part of medicine's unknowns, the consequences are twofold. One is the disproportionate pain and death caused in a vast portion of the population. The other is more existential, in that it undermines many people's sense of knowing their own bodies, and so also how much they trust themselves. Another tragedy that results from the prejudices and gender stereotypes driving medicine, for me, is that in trying to render the supposedly impenetrable female body penetrable, it has rendered me impenetrable to myself.

I was raised in a medical family and received extensive biology lessons throughout school. And yet still, I wasn't sure about my body. When medical procedures felt wrong, when what medical professionals were telling me felt wrong, I always felt that, given medicine's authority, it must be my own sense of self that was misguided. I blamed my body for not fitting the tools that medicine used, rather than questioning why those tools were not designed for me. It took learning about how societal power imbalances shape the ideas we hold about bodies for me to understand that there could be another way, that there was a version of medicine that could prioritise different interests; that I could expect more.

Let's return to that image of female musculature. A small disclaimer: the picture is actually not strictly of musculature but of milk ducts, and many individuals, scientists and otherwise, were quick to make this point online when they responded to the picture's hype, adamant that their male default was simply more accurate. Only, that depends on what accurate means here: what are we trying to accurately represent?

Medicine has formed its image of the body based on the structures and systems that matter to male bodies. In order to understand female bodies, medicine will need to shapeshift as much as the bodies it thinks it knows. The boundaries between fields will fade as their tools and facts merge to address female-specific questions. Here, from a female biology perspective, it makes sense to include milk ducts in diagrams of musculature due to the role that tissue stimulation plays in releasing the hormone oxytocin which activates the mammary muscles to eject milk.

In other words, musculature needs milk ducts.

In this book I want to tell the story of how women have been excluded from science, not only in terms of underrepresentation in numbers but more insidiously, through the long-held ideas that can often seem intuitive but are based on misguided science which in turn also misguides our understanding of the female body.

I want to explain those feelings of disconnect I have often felt in the doctor's consultation room, and my own preoccupation with a body that always seemed not just my responsibility but also my failure.

I want to expose the ideas driving a male-centric version of medicine and medical practise and point to alternatives. Ideas are powerful tools, and by claiming them, we can advance the cause of women's health.

I want to share the magical potential science holds to change the world we know.

Good feminism is good science – and good science is good for us all.

PART 1

Inconceivable Bodies

As far as medicine is concerned, a woman's life starts when her period does and ends when she gives birth. This narrow definition emanates from that close association between women and childbearing, so close that her body disappears into her womb, has become synonymous with her reproductive potential. But this reproductive timeline misses almost everything. It even fails to encompass the full scope of factors contributing to a woman's reproductive health. It has limited the medical attention women get and the questions scientists have deigned to ask about their bodies. It has sustained that toxic silence around the unexplained illnesses and problems women experience throughout their lives, when these haven't mapped onto the 'natural', neatly contained timeline of the 'quintessential' female.

Gynaecology is an area where we see the gendered ideas about women in focus, because this field is 'all about women'. Only it isn't. Femininity has always been fraught, with conflicting demands placed on individuals, like the imperative to be both virginal and sexy; an impossible, contradictory ideal that has been mobilised throughout history to silence and stifle and torment women. On an individual level, upholding womanhood has always been a losing battle. It has always meant suffering, remaining silent about the parts of ourselves that undermine our pristine facades. The same is true of femininity in science and medicine, with doctors rejecting the issues that don't pertain to childbirth, or don't register as 'sexy', and with women dismissing their own experiences when these don't align with what they perceive to be the 'natural' female experience – be that the life-inhibiting discomfort of uterine prolapse, the mental health complications following childbirth, or physiological responses to sexual arousal that, we think, we are told, science can't explain.

As we begin to unpick the issues that really matter to female health in the areas of gynaecology, obstetrics, sexology and hormones, we will start to push against the boundaries of that biological (aka reproductive) timeline that constricts us. We will start to see a blurring of lines, then a flow of unruly menstrual blood that takes us to new places, other areas of health, that connect gynaecology to other areas of medicine and also show us how we might do medicine differently; might rethink the boundaries of its fields, the way care is implemented, and the meaning of its concepts, including gender. This kind of imagination is dangerous, it's bold and, often, it's tantalisingly simple. Once we can think about our lifelines beyond the shackles of a skewed interpretation of our biology, potential treatments begin to present themselves; glaringly obvious. The solutions to women's health problems don't seem so inconceivable after all.

Chapter 1

The Gynaecological Way of Life

When I was eighteen, I started taking the pill. I didn't have a regular sex life, but I aspired to have one soon. I was dating a boy and it was heading that way and I knew that I had to be 'safe'. That meant not getting an STD and not getting pregnant. But the real reason I wanted to start taking oral contraceptives was that I wanted to be like the cool girls at school. The girls who popped the pills from their neon packaging (as the boys watched), at the same time, every day. It was a rite of passage, a ritual that made you desirable, because you were announcing your desire. These girls were confident – I recognised empowerment before I ever knew the word. They were *real* women. And I wanted to be a woman. Ergo, I had to take the pill.

Only my body and mind couldn't handle these heights of emancipation. I felt bloated, swollen, I felt like crying a lot of the time, my periods had gone from trickles to heavy flows. My own body was unrecognisable to me – it scared me.

I went to the doctor who told me girls often reacted to the pill in these ways. I asked what I could do and was told I had to live with the side effects. Or stop. The medication was what it was – standard, largely effective. It was my body that had failed to respond. They couldn't tell me why. Silently, I stopped taking my oral contraceptive. I wouldn't be having sex for a while anyway. So, I watched the cool girls pop their pills and felt like I'd never know how it felt to be a *real woman*.

Looking back, I wonder how much of those other girls' bravado hid their own discomfort. If I carried the social pressure I felt on my body in silence, perhaps they did too. If I kept my body's unruliness a secret, perhaps their bodies also rebelled behind closed doors. Perhaps they also blamed their bodies, rather than an inhumane culture, when they didn't conform. Gynaecology had let us down. And given the general neglect of the medical field that is supposed to support our reproductive health, it would make sense that the majority of women felt as I did then.

For an area supposedly so defining of female biology, gynaecology has been ferociously neglected. And with less than 2.1% of publicly funded research being dedicated solely to women's reproductive health, the conversations within medicine are as limited as they are in society at large. This silence is dangerous for women. Where knowledge is lacking, harmful ideas about both women and our bodies fill the gaps.

This silent incubator for stigma disempowers women in our reproductive health. Some 31% of women in the UK have experienced severe reproductive health symptoms in the last year, ranging from heavy menstrual bleeding to menopause, and infertility.[1] Less than half of these women seek help, regardless of the severity of their symptoms, and most cite the stigma surrounding reproductive health as the key inhibiting factor. That means that in the UK, over 15% of women go unheard and untreated. And the women who do puncture through this fear of their supposedly unruly bodies in order to get the medical help they need are often met with silence.

Journalist Lynn Enright relied not just on research but also on her personal experience with unmet gynaecological needs to write her book, *Vagina: A Re-education*[2], having had her searing monthly pain dismissed. It turned out to be a uterine fibroid. Even following a hysteroscopy to examine the inside of Enright's womb, doctors were unable to explain her condition. The problem then is not just that women don't report symptoms – an issue that happens for a number of reasons – it is also a lack of medical knowledge that helps sustain a taboo around gynaecological issues. This means that even when women raise concerns, they are often met with blank stares from doctors.

Where does this silence in medicine come from? According to Andrew Horne, Professor of Gynaecology and Reproductive Sciences at the University of Edinburgh, it is because the decision makers in medicine struggle as much with the stigma around reproductive health as the patients themselves. The decision-making panels of big funding bodies, such as the Medical Research Council, the US National Institutes of Health and the Wellcome Trust, have historically been dominated by men. Thus, when research related to gynaecology or obstetrics was proposed, it would have struck many of the panellists, who would not have had first-hand experience with these problems, as subsidiary, awkward and/or trivial. As a result, a lot of funding went to conditions that affected just men or were cross gender. Consider diabetes – it affects one in ten women, the same ratio as endometriosis, a condition where tissue similar to the lining of the womb grows in other places, such as the ovaries and fallopian tubes, potentially causing painful periods, chronic pelvic pain, painful sex and painful bowel movements, as well as potential fertility problems. While the impact on quality of life is considered to be similar in these diseases, the proportion of funding that goes towards treating diabetes is around twenty times more than the amount of funding that goes towards treating endometriosis.[3]

Besides government funding bodies, charities may offer an alternative route to funding for researchers. But there are very few charities dedicated solely to female reproductive health compared to, for example, cardiovascular disease. The British Heart Foundation invests an average of £100 million a year; Cancer Research UK funded £455 million worth of research from 2019 to 2020. Now compare that to the mere £975,000 spent on research by Wellbeing of Women, one of the few charities dedicated solely to female reproductive health research in the UK. As one of few of its kind, the charity's support is high in demand and in 2019, only 11% of all applications considered by its research advisory committee were funded – Cancer Research UK approved 28% of research applications in the same period.

If we were to compare these figures directly, the discrepancy would be glaring – the point is, we never do. A comparison implies that the fields are, indeed, comparable; that gynaecology is on a par with the likes of cancer research in terms of scientific credibility, as well as importance to human health. Yet the specialisation of funding bodies, along with disciplines, means that governments and board members don't often take this holistic view. This kind of sustained myopia is one of the most frustrating and infuriating obstacles to medicine reform because it blocks the possibility of discussion.

Professor Horne is one of the lucky few who made a successful application to Wellbeing of Women. He spoke to me from his clinic, tired, it seemed, but pragmatic about the challenges he and his field faced. In the often-demoralising funding environment for female chronic reproductive conditions, researchers like Horne have had to find ways to innovate. Horne is investigating how anti-cancer drugs can be repurposed to treat endometriosis. This means that the sometimes decade's worth of investments put into cancer drugs that don't make it to market – sums that wouldn't be available in the field of women's health specifically – don't go to waste.

Endometriosis remains an enigmatic disease, its origins still unknown, and debate reigns on how best to treat it. It impacts severely on the lives of sufferers: around 40% said they were concerned about losing their job due to their struggles with the symptoms of the disease; two in five teenagers missed school and exams. And while 1.5 million women and people in the UK suffer from endometriosis, the average diagnosis time is eight years and that hasn't improved in a decade.[4] As Lone Hummelshoj, Chief Executive of the World Endometriosis Research Foundation, puts it, 'the minute you say menstruation [women's health] gets dismissed'.[5]

Stigma doesn't only block research into gynaecology and obstetrics, it prevents existing knowledge from being properly implemented too. I spoke to Professor Lesley Regan, President of the Royal College of Obstetricians and Gynaecologists (RCOG), who emphasised how we can powerfully enhance the wellbeing of women by taking their needs seriously and responding with simple changes in the delivery of care. She gave the example of the response to cervical cancer. There are highly effective preventative screening programmes available that have the potential to prevent 70% of cervical cancer deaths. Cervical screening, or a smear test, involves swabbing cells from the cervix, which are then sent to a laboratory to identify any abnormal cells that could lead to cervical cancer. Since 1988, the UK has led a centrally organised NHS cervical screening programme. This programme draws on a population-based registry to reach all women within the screening age range (twenty to sixty-four years), a systematic process of call and recall, national coordination and quality assurance.

The cervical screening programme is estimated to save around 5,000 lives each year, yet the number of women attending screenings has fluctuated over time, rather than simply trending upwards. As is the case with many female-specific conditions, celebrity endorsement has gone some way to raising awareness. The reality TV star Jade Goody, who died from cervical cancer in 2009, became a public advocate for smear tests. Following Goody's diagnosis, and after her death, NHS figures showed that half-a-million more women booked a smear test.[6] But these numbers soon declined. In fact, the uptake of these programmes declined consistently between 2015 and 2019, hitting a twenty-year low. A celebrity's endorsement, effective as it can be in the moment, can only paper over the cracks in a system in which women do not feel willing or able to attend their screenings. One woman in three does not attend. The number of deaths from cervical cancer has been predicted to grow by 143% between 2015 and 2040. Professor Regan said that when these statistics were presented to the Chief Medical Officer (CMO), they asked, 'For which country is this?', expecting the numbers to reflect somewhere less economically developed or somewhere with a lack of resources. Yet these appalling statistics reveal the complacency of a country that has all the resources it needs yet has failed to understand what prevents women from accessing them.

Research into the reasons for missed screenings revealed that, among other reasons, fear, embarrassment and cultural barriers prevent women from attending. This research has been slow to emerge in a culture where the tendency is to discard women's feelings as irrational while placing blame on women, rather than on the healthcare system, for failing to accommodate them.

One of the silver linings for women of the coronavirus pandemic was that with additional barriers to regular healthcare appointments, a new endeavour was launched in the form of at-home testing in the UK. In a trial, over 31,000 women, all at least six months overdue for a test, will be posted or given an at-home sampling kit by their GP, allowing them to take the swab in the privacy and convenience of their own home. This self-sampling method addresses a long-standing problem in the care for women, by taking their experiences seriously and responding with a change in testing to suit *them*. This shows the power of listening to women and responding to their needs.

At-home testing is just one example of the simple measures Professor Regan and the RCOG have proposed in their *Better for Women* report to improve the health and wellbeing of girls and women. Beyond standalone interventions in reproductive care, they argue that we need to rethink how we manage women's health much more holistically, and that this provides a model for healthcare delivery in general; a system of care that emphasises health enhancement over disease intervention. Changes are urgently needed across the board in delivering reproductive care to women. In Professor Regan's words: 'There is so much more to women's health than becoming pregnant and delivering a healthy baby. There is a whole life course to consider.'[7]

As my own introduction into the world of contraception attests, we need tailored support from a much earlier age; we need to understand how gynaecological issues affect other aspects of our health; we need to have informed, open conversations about the considerations – social and medical – that come into play when making these choices. Treating women for pregnancy-related complications after the fact is just a glimmer in a prism of the integrated medical and psychological and social systems that make a woman's life. And looking through this prism will not just show us a new way of enhancing the quality of life for women, but reveal new scientific questions that span disparate fields, and perhaps also a new way of practising medicine altogether.

This approach won't come easy. The fact that many of the social solutions seem simple may make them less likely to be taken seriously – we have certainly seen evidence of this throughout history. It will mean a radical shift from the way women have been treated in gynaecology and beyond. For most of history, women's health has been centred around the ability to bear children. Far from being patients to be treated, women have been seen as vessels, their health only useful in that it was essential to the delivering of a healthy baby. In obstetrics, this meant that doctors would refrain from treating a mother for fear of harming the foetus. Other aspects of a woman's health beyond the parameters of childbearing simply fell outside of the doctor's remit, and well beyond the limited timeframe of care. For many of these problems, including pre-eclampsia (a pregnancy disorder characterised by high blood pressure that increases the risk of poor outcomes for both mother and baby) and gestational diabetes, it has long been an adage in obstetrics that 'childbirth is the cure', meaning that once the baby is born, the issue with the mother's body is no longer a medical problem. Thus the health of the mother only matters as a means to ensuring the health of her child. In reality, women who have suffered pre-eclampsia often experience heart disease and stroke in middle age, and those with gestational diabetes have an increased risk of Type 2 diabetes later in life. These gestational syndromes actually irreversibly, in some cases, change a mother's physiology, unmasking a vulnerability to future disease. Understanding this means that research can be done to identify risk factors in mothers, and to plan preventative treatment after they've given birth. Caring for women has to be so much more than purely treatment relating to the baby.

Obstetrics and gynaecology are by-products of the idea that a woman is a childbearing body, and nothing more. Once pregnancy is completed, medicine steps away, and a woman's body is once again rendered invisible in a male-centric system. The point is not that the understanding of women's bodies through childbirth developed in these fields is unimportant, but that we cannot stop there. Knowledge about women's bodies through pregnancy presents a valuable resource in the form of a set of prompts that should push doctors and scientists to investigate and pre-empt the impact of pregnancy on all dimensions of health across a lifespan. These fields need to be drawn out and drawn upon to bust open the doors of fields formed around the needs of male bodies, to grow a new integrated form of medicine that takes into account the entirety of a woman – her body and her life – and not just one small slice of her.

That's why we need a lifespan approach – a new way of planning healthcare that aims to ensure that women's health and wellbeing over the course of their entire lives – not just their reproductive health during pregnancy – are prioritised. This may sound like quite the undertaking, but all that is actually required is better organisation. As Professor Regan's report says, this 'can be achieved by placing women and their predictable needs at the centre of our service planning and taking some simple practical steps to harness existing resources and use them more efficiently'. Recommendations include providing easy access to contraception, including postpartum. This intervention is also key because the abortion rate is rising, predominantly among older women who don't have access to reliable long-acting reversible contraception (LARC). That suggestion may seem blindingly obvious but has yet to be inserted into medical care.

Another recommendation focuses on learning from indicators in the reproductive years to influence future health. This includes, for example, collecting data on general health and lifestyle habits before, during and after pregnancy to identify possible future health issues. It also states the importance of ensuring that data transfers between the place of birth and primary care services. The six-week postnatal GP check that is standard in the UK could in this way offer an important opportunity to identify women at risk from mental or physical health issues. Currently, time pressure and inconsistent training means this check-up is a missed opportunity. In all of these cases, simple, often bureaucratic changes could ensure that a woman's health is finally treated across a life and not just the span of a pregnancy.

We shouldn't, of course, even need to persuade people to care about women's health outside the areas of gynaecology and obstetrics. But given that this seems to be the task before

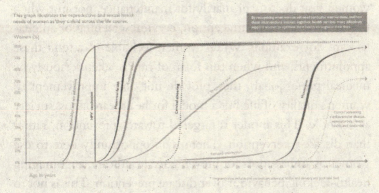

This graph illustrates the lifespan approach to reproductive
and sexual healthcare of women. Interventions at
predictable and crucial points in a woman's biological life
help to optimise her health and prevent disease.[8]

us, what makes the case for this approach especially persuasive
– aside from basic decency – is that international evidence has
shown that healthy women are the cornerstone of healthy
societies.[9] While women make up 51% of the population, they
represent a much higher proportion of the primary carers in
society and so exert a strong influence on the health behaviours of their families and local communities. In other words,
the health of one woman goes on to have a ripple effect that
extends much, much further beyond the confines of just her
own body. The basic truth is, in the long term, it makes sense
both financially and societally to care about women's health.
(Since the Better for Women report was published, major
progress has been made with the announcement of the first
Women's Health Strategy for England, with Professor Dame
Regan as its Ambassador, which builds on the report's recommendations.) As if we needed more convincing.

Professor Regan also reiterated how important it is that

women visit doctors primarily for maintenance, not just when they're unwell, for contraception, cervical screening or antenatal care, for example. When women feel able to attend these appointments, and when this form of care is taken seriously by medical professionals, they provide not only improvement to women's quality of life but a model for healthcare across society as a whole. This model is targeted towards prevention, rather than disease intervention. There is an opportunity here to use women as ambassadors for preventative healthcare, encouraging health-seeking behaviour over disease prevention. This is not to hold women responsible or to demand more invisible labour from them in a society where they already tend to be the unpaid caregivers, but to develop a system that supports them and their needs, thereby cultivating a form of healthcare that is better for everyone. To do this effectively means asking women about their experiences, listening to women and making their words count. It sounds so simple. And yet . . .

So, when I decided to take the pill – for so many reasons, but mainly because I'd internalised lessons about what safe sex meant – I thought the process would be simple. There was a defined problem with a straightforward solution. Except the solution wasn't straightforward. My body didn't respond the way that medicine's idea of a passively responsive, generic body of a woman should. Medicine couldn't tell me why or offer me alternatives and so it wasn't solving *my* problem. Medicine got the answer wrong because it got the problem wrong.

For me, and probably a lot of women like me, taking the pill was about so much more than 'safe sex'. It was about making a decision about and for my own body and feeling confident, secure and empowered in that decision. In the moments that I relied on medicine to do that it often fell short. If medicine had dared to complicate its tidy solutions with questions about the priorities and needs of women themselves, if it had acknowledged its shortcomings, perhaps I would have felt less like a failure of a woman and instead pointed a finger at an institution that was failing to meet my needs.

Taking the pill, to me, was a watershed moment. But what happens when those moments don't go according to plan? When we, as individuals and individual bodies, don't conform to the generic course of the life we thought we were meant to live? Perhaps we only recognise these moments in hindsight. We look back and think, 'Oh yes, that's when I became aware of the femaleness of my body', or, 'Now I see that's when I first felt my body wasn't enough.' Medicine needs its own watershed moment too. And its new geography might look very different – sprawling, unruly, leading us through the course of a life and between generations – but it will be more habitable for more people. Not just the 49% – although, in the end, it will be better for them too.

Medical professionals need to talk to women. They need to be guided by those conversations as they interrogate their assumptions about what female bodies need. This requires that medicine mobilises its knowledge in new ways across disciplines and across a woman's entire lifespan. But breaking the silence on women's reproductive health has implications for medicine as a whole. For a while, we'll hear a messy cacophony of experiences, perhaps contradictory but all united in the challenge they pose to a supposedly streamlined system of diagnoses and cures, to a discipline that is meant to reassure us that it has all the answers. Yet this has always been a façade: behind it were women in pain.

Thus, medicine will need to lose itself to find itself. But breaking through the stigma around female reproductive health, for one, will reveal the varied ways in which gynaecology factors into women's lives, creating fertile ground for a discipline that is not only effective but also cares.

Chapter 2

Sexy Research

Across the board, whether we are looking at policymakers, funding panels or scientists themselves, the stigma around gynaecology and obstetrics is kept alive by a collective of individuals who, whether consciously or not, seem to want to keep these female-centred fields at arm's length.

In science, where scientists rely on grants with an interest in their subject area to fund their research, the lack of money being funnelled into gynaecology and obstetrics begins to explain why these might be less appealing to researchers who will anticipate difficulty in funding their work. Yet the issue is (at least) two-fold. Many researchers in the field agree that a lack of funding isn't actually the primary concern. Professor David Williams, the Independent Chair at Wellbeing of Women, confirmed that there is in fact substantial funding, provided by the National Institute for Health and Care Research (NIHR), the Medical Research Council (MRC) and the Wellcome Trust, going into his field of birth and pregnancy research. So if the problem is not the availability of funds full stop, what is it?

Professor Williams has highlighted a deeper, much more pervasive issue: the general discomfort extending beyond silences on funding boards to the medical professionals themselves, which makes these important areas of research less appealing to scientists deciding on a specialism in the first place. Williams, who specialises in clinical care and research for pregnant women with acute or chronic medical disorders, described to me how these areas aren't considered 'sexy'. It's a turn of phrase easily misconstrued in gynaecology, but what the professor is talking about is the unfortunate fact, pervasive across science, that certain fields are considered much more exciting by new researchers, because certain types of scientific advancement are valued more highly than others.

We see this across the board in scientific research. Sending a rover to Mars is far more exciting than monitoring background radiation. Discovering a new species is more exciting than doing conservation work. Developing an RNA-based COVID vaccine is more exciting than developing a system to distribute it. The areas that are the most appealing for budding researchers and scientists are those that hold the potential for 'high-tech' and 'ground-breaking' types of discovery. The kinds of discoveries that get you into headlines, merit an OBE or lead to a film based on your research.

Professor Williams pointed to the Human papillomavirus (HPV) vaccine as an example of the kind of exciting work in which researchers want to be involved. While the HPV vaccine, to you, may not seem glitzy and exciting, it's important to bear in mind that before the early aughts, nobody had heard of it. And then, all of a sudden, it was propelled to stardom. Introduced in 2006, this vaccine to treat cancer was a total gamechanger.

HPV is a group of over 200 viruses that are very common in humans. The virus infects the skin and cells lining the inside of the body. Most types do not cause any problems, however almost all cases of cervical cancer are caused by HPV. The HPV vaccine was first developed at the University of Queensland, Australia, by Professors Ian Frazer and Jian Zhou and released in the US in 2006 to tackle the, at the time, highly prevalent incidence of cervical cancer. By the following year, the vaccine had been approved in eighty countries, including Australia and across the European Union. As of October 2019, 100 countries worldwide are vaccinating against HPV, and the World Health Organization (WHO) now recommends HPV vaccines as part of routine vaccinations in all countries. As a result, there has been an over 80% reduction in HPV among sixteen-to-twenty-one-year-old women.[1]

Ironically – though perhaps not surprisingly – even in this technically advanced branch of reproductive science, the German virologist Harald zur Hausen, who identified the role of HPV in cervical cancer that later formed the basis for the vaccine, had his own proposals rejected by pharmaceutical companies who believed the vaccine would not be profitable. Nonetheless, just over two decades later, after the vaccine was finally developed, zur Hausen was awarded the 2008 Nobel Prize in medicine for his discoveries. This is the kind of science that researchers are remembered for. And this is the kind of science that many new researchers look to as an example of what they might go on to achieve.

While the vaccine has undoubtedly been a major break-through in the prevention of cancer in girls and women, the glorification of these one-off achievements has left other important areas in obstetrics and gynaecology comparatively neglected. Other avenues of scientific research might not hold promise of individual acclaim because they may rely on collaboration. They might not go down in history as life-saving interventions because they may tackle medical conditions that aren't life-threatening but that do ruin lives. Many of these are termed 'invisible' diseases. Chronic conditions like endometriosis, as I've already discussed, or pelvic pain and heavy menstrual bleeding, seriously interfere in a woman's ability to function at school, at work and in intimate relationships. These conditions impact throughout lives and may cause serious harm if left untreated, but women are often able to hide them – or feel they have to – to get through the day. In other words, these conditions aren't sexy. Which means that the work and research done to relieve these conditions aren't sexy either.

While cancer has seen the introduction of the HPV vaccine, improved screening, treatment and even cures over the past years, life-inhibiting conditions in female gynaecology have often been deemed much less interesting to researchers.

Stigma around women's health only begins to explain the lack of research on obstetrics and gynaecology. There is also the equally sexist issue around the perception of which problems are deemed 'sexy', meaning that scientifically advanced breakthrough research is prioritised over the important research that will enhance the lives of women in the long term. Having more female researchers driving forward research will undoubtedly help redefine what is considered 'sexy' science and may even help spur on a much-needed destigmatisation of the women's health issues that this research might tackle. In truth, some of the most ground-breaking advances in women's health will come from asking questions and listening to women, and responding with pragmatic, often low-tech solutions.

Midwifery and research

Some of the most important research on the long-term well-being of women following pregnancy and childbirth is being done by midwives. This is because midwives tend to conduct research into the lived experiences of individual women going through pregnancy and childbirth. Some of this information has had a big impact in recent years.

The UK has one of the highest rates of preterm and stillbirths in the developed world, along with maternity services that cost the most money in medical negligence claims and the second highest rate of claims. I shouldn't have been surprised when Dr James Harris, a senior clinical lecturer in evidence-based midwifery, told me on a mid-pandemic Zoom call, that an intervention that reduces preterm births by 24% and makes women 16% less likely to lose their baby, while also greatly increasing satisfaction in services, does already exist.[2] The brutal truth is if it were a medicine, everyone would be taking it; if it were a piece of technology, every hospital would have one. Yet, this intervention is not a cutting-edge vaccine so it's not in general use. What it does is so simple – ensuring continuity of the midwife who cares for a pregnant woman from the beginning of pregnancy to the point when she is discharged postnatally.[3]

Multiple randomised controlled trials and reviews have demonstrated the benefits of this continuity of care, yet only a small minority of women receive their care in this way. This is especially concerning because this service model most benefits vulnerable and at risk families, where an ongoing relationship means a midwife is more attuned to their particular needs.[4]

'If this was a treatment that fixed erectile dysfunction, if this cured prostate cancer,' Dr Harris laments, 'there wouldn't have been this kind of delay in implementing it into general care.' I find myself nodding furiously as I listen. This is all familiar territory: how many more TV ads have I watched claiming to solve a man's erectile dysfunction than ones offering help to women for their endometriosis?

To explain this lag, Dr Harris points to an ongoing distrust among government decision makers, scientists and medical practitioners, of non-pharmaceutical or non-technical medical solutions. These studies into the real experiences of women propose solutions that rely on the strength of relationships, of trust-building between midwives and pregnant women over time. And these studies take time to do. They aren't the silver-bullet solutions symptomatic of so-called sexy research and so aren't considered as scientific.

Dr Harris gives us another example of how a male-dominated research culture, out of touch with the experienced reality of women's medical conditions, prioritises research questions that it answers with high-tech solutions, and thereby also prioritises a competitive race to scientific acclaim over the wellbeing of the female patients the field is supposed to benefit. In 2017, NHS England finally began to implement the continuity of carer model as proposed by the midwives through the Maternity Transformation Programme.[5] The aim was initially that 20% of women would receive care in this way, and to increase this to 35% by 2020, although the coronavirus pandemic somewhat derailed these plans. Nonetheless, this policy drive makes the potential impact of this study big, comparable even, when you take into account the long-term health of the mothers and their children, to the reach of the HPV vaccine. This is the first time that midwifery research has impacted government policy in the UK.

Despite these moves towards what is really just more patient-centric research in obstetrics, the temptation to look for the most scientifically advanced and immediate solutions to medical problems, rather than measures that benefit the long-term health of women's bodies, prevails. Dr Harris points to the research on the coronavirus funded in the UK as a case in point. The money here went to treatments for the condition. With ten licensed vaccines at the time of writing, and more on the way, comparatively little funding has gone to research on long COVID, on coping with life after a serious viral disease – or indeed coping with the fallout society has experienced while merely trying to get through the pandemic.[6]

Dr Harris is particularly concerned by the lack of research on the psychological impact of being locked in as a new mother. COVID has seen drastic changes to the maternity services offered in England. Most maternity units removed the option of homebirth as it was felt that this would be unsafe, given that the ambulance service could not guarantee collection within five minutes of an emergency call to get to a hospital. This was devastating for many mothers. Additionally, new mothers couldn't have their partners with them for scans, so many fathers didn't see or hear their babies until they were born, and many women were told about their miscarriages without a support person present. There is very little research funded by medical charities to explore the long-term societal and psychological effects of these short-term emergency measures. No one is asking, for example, how it has impacted maternal–foetal attachment or the bonding between the mother and her new child. While retrospective studies have interviewed women, very few have asked how we might prospectively improve the mental wellbeing of these mothers.

Slowly, awareness is growing in the medical community around the need for research into the psychological and social dimensions of medical care in obstetrics. Research policy bodies have urged the funders that we have seen are the drivers of research to prioritise women's reproductive health. These investigations have, in particular, homed in on the important and neglected area of pregnancy and mental health.[7] While depression and anxiety are the most common mental health problems during pregnancy, affecting 15–20% of women in the first year after childbirth,[8] only 4% of pregnancy research funding goes to this area.

Mental health during and after pregnancy presents scientists and medical professionals with a complex and multi-factorial problem. Mothers face an increased risk of depression after giving birth, partly due to any medical issues that might arise in the third trimester of pregnancy, but also due to previous mental health conditions, as well as various social and environmental factors during pregnancy and after giving birth, from mother–baby bonding to the drugs administered, to addressing pre-standing mental health issues. Yet while the causes are multiple and require disentangling from one another, solutions are already available. They aren't scientifically advanced but simply require better organisation. Often, evidence-based practice standards exist yet aren't implemented in clinics.[9] This less scientifically 'exciting' solution has once again attracted less attention from funders who like to invest in sexy science. This response won't be based on a single cure but on ongoing support. 'Process', as a concept, is not acknowledged in the valuation of scientific careers and isn't valued by funders. Yet 'process', rather than 'cure', is what differentiates between good and substandard care.

It is important to emphasise that this sexy science approach doesn't only limit the care available to women. It is detrimental to everyone. This model, so prevalent in the medical world, that looks for so-called elegant, one-stop solutions to diseases with singular, curable causes, limits how far scientists delve in their understanding and how far medical professionals go in supporting patients. Take erectile dysfunction as a corollary in men. The pharmaceutical company Pfizer introduced the drug Viagra in the late 1990s for what had until then been a normal aspect of aging or a physiological response to a normal range of emotions. Viagra was initially prescribed for erectile dysfunction due to medical issues such as diabetes and spinal cord damage, but was transformed by the company into a product sold to any man to enhance his ability to achieve an erection for a longer period of time. By medicalising erectile dysfunction, Pfizer also asserted and spread, through extensive marketing campaigns, a presumed standard of sexual performance, implying that anything that fell short of this standard was pathological and caused mental harm. The question here is how much harm Pfizer has done by asserting a sexual standard that never before existed by proposing a streamlined cure to a debatable problem. Rather than investigating how men actually feel about erectile dysfunction – and it isn't as bad as you might think[10] – a culture and economy of medicine that values a cutting-edge 'fix', a simple, streamlined pill, over messy, complicated, culturally dependent, individualised care, have emerged. And this culture doesn't just fail to treat problems; it creates new ones too.

In the areas of pregnancy and mental health, as in gynaecology, but also, as we'll see later, in cardiology and bone research, much of the knowledge and resources needed to provide care to women already exist. Medicine simply needs to harness the full scope of both medical and experiential knowledge to deliver the best care to women. No single field can offer the tools needed to care for women's reproductive health; how could it, when the specialties in medicine have formed around the questions that matter most to (often male) researchers, rather than female biology? The challenge here may lie not in technological innovation but in inventing equally impressive tools for collaboration across fields or for gauging and responding to the needs of patients in medicine. Perhaps it is time for a Nobel Prize for social rather than scientific innovation in medical research.

Chapter 3

'Wellness' and 'Empowerment'

When I was twenty-five, I discovered conversations I'd never known existed. It was 2017, I was at university, and it felt like suddenly women's reproductive health wasn't taboo anymore. After a childhood of forceful silent messages, of shame and of feeling alone in my aloneness in the medical system, a gust of empowerment seemed to have blown the roof off that isolating silo.

Perhaps it was also the university climate, the fact that I was studying topics like reproductive rights and was surrounded by feminists. Perhaps it was just that I was older, sexually active, the childish giddiness around the topic gradually subsiding. Whatever it was, women's reproductive health now was not just an acceptable topic worthy of conversation, it was hot.

There were articles, there were videos, there were products, all of which promised me liberation and a deeper understanding of my own biology. Some promised me control over my periods, better sex, some even offered me solutions to problems I never knew I had.

Vaginas could be dirty, I was told, could suffer from odours that needed cleaning. Vaginas could get saggy, I learnt, requiring exercises to keep them tight and young. It was refreshing, this newfound openness about my most private parts, splashed across the pages of *Glamour* magazine, or even in 'high-brow' sources, like *The Times*. But it slowly became overwhelming. That familiar pang returned of not being woman-enough, of being abnormal, deficient, *dirty*. I had traded in one form of shame for another. And now I knew it was all my responsibility.

My vulva (that was the word, I learnt, for the female external genitals, not *vagina* which refers to the tube connecting the external genitals to the cervix of the uterus), my newfound educational material had taught me, required upkeep. Along with emancipation, it seemed, came expectations: 'cleanliness', tightness, an absence of any smell. And along with these expectations came shame when I didn't, couldn't meet them. It didn't occur to me to question whose expectations these were.

In 2017, just as I was discovering these new dimensions to the labour of being a woman, gynaecologist Dr Jen Gunter rose to viral fame when she clashed with celebrity Gwyneth Paltrow over the recommendation made by Paltrow's lifestyle and wellness e-commerce company, Goop. So began Dr Gunter's war on wellness – an industry now worth more than $4.2tn (£3.5tn) and almost overnight, she became the world's most famous gynaecologist.

In response to so many people asking her about them, Dr Gunter wrote an open letter to Paltrow[1] about the jade eggs or 'vaginal rocks' that Goop sold, promising that they would 'balance' one's menstrual cycle and 'intensify feminine energy', among other things. All were presented as medically necessary upkeep and part of a modern woman's self-care regime.

Paltrow once called the vagina a 'cultural firestorm',[2] although this is mainly true of her own. Paltrow's reproductive system has birthed not only markets for the smell of her nether regions in candle form but a veritable movement around the revival of historical health hacks, such as the ancient practice of vaginal steaming or the esoteric mysticism of a compound she calls 'sex dust'. Not to mention the 2020 Netflix documentary that follows the Goop team as they discover an array of what could most generously be described as 'alternative' medical interventions but perhaps more realistically as unsubstantiated, dangerous and harmful gambles with human health.

In her letter to Paltrow, Dr Gunter took issue with the various scientific inaccuracies around the description of the jade eggs on Goop's website: 'the claim that they can balance hormones', for example, was biologically impossible. Indeed, Dr Gunter's criticisms were echoed in a 2018 $145,000 lawsuit brought by California's consumer protection office. Goop paid the fine, but continues to sell the eggs, albeit alongside a slightly modified, much more modest, description of their wide-ranging potential.

While the law stepped in to confirm that jade eggs really couldn't balance hormones, Dr Gunter's critique went beyond the science. In her letter, she also took issue more generally with the messages Goop was sending out about a warped form of female gynaecological empowerment.

> My issue begins with the very start of your post on jade eggs, specifically that 'queens and concubines used them to stay in shape for emperors.' Nothing says female empowerment more than the only reason to do this is for your man!

However misguided though, perhaps it is the brand of 'empowerment' that Goop sells that explains its commercial success. Perhaps what appeals is that through Goop's apparent celebration of female energy and promises of orgasm, it offers the assurance that through a more positive relationship with our bodies, vagina owners may experience the medical benefits they've been unable to access elsewhere, and so may gain control over their own biology. Is it perhaps telling that many of the techniques now resurfacing on the websites of brands like Goop originate from 1970s' feminist manuals, written by women who similarly placed little faith in the medical institution to care for their bodies?

In the absence of a medical gynaecology that responds to their needs, perhaps it is no wonder that women have returned to the vaginal mythology of yesteryear to recapture a sense of agency over their health. When female health was deemed unsexy and pushed to the sidelines and women's reports on their health were not worth listening to, is it any surprise that the wellness industry stepped in to offer an alternative? Or that some of us may have been all too eager to accept the new messaging without examining it too closely, in want of a solution to unheard problems? To anything that might offer help?

Dr Gunter has noted how Goop, and other wellbeing brands like it, exacerbate the discomfort women might feel when talking about gynaecological issues, promoting a 'clean' version of female biology that is dependent on purchasable products to manage a reproductive system that is otherwise inherently seen as dirty. In the first anti-Goop post Dr Gunter wrote, back in 2015, she took on vaginal steaming, recommended by the brand as a next-level detox, once again to 'balance female hormone levels'. Dr Gunter made the point that vaginal steaming is: a) unnecessary, as the vagina and uterus and vulva are all self-cleaning; and b) harmful to the environment needed for the lactobacilli that keep vaginas healthy.

The technique of vaginal steaming itself – a process whereby you squat over a container of often herbal-infused steam that wafts upwards into your vagina – is tied to the historical belief that women are unclean inside. It dates back to ancient Greece, when it was believed that the womb wandered the body causing disease and could be coaxed back, like an animal, by putting fragrant herbs between the legs. Academic and popular thought built on this idea, further entrenching the view, considered scientifically proven by the late nineteenth century, that women were at the mercy of their biology, and so were mentally and physically inferior and unfit to participate in public life.

Yet this concept of the toxic uterus, integral to a patriarchal medical tradition, has somehow re-emerged under the guise of female empowerment. It has slipped into our lives as inconspicuously as a jade egg. At the core of Goop's health agenda is a general fear of femininity, a need to suppress and control it, by mobilising old, patriarchal biological myths.

That it is not only bad science, but bad feminism too.

Goop's health agenda leads to pressure to perform a sexualised version of femininity. This idea of female health is not based on what women want or what feels good or what is healthy but on what is deemed 'sexy' by a pseudo-feminist culture that carries physically and psychologically harmful messages.

GripTok, Kegels, empowerment and wellness

My life went on, magazines and newspapers gave way to TikTok, which I found, one afternoon in my late twenties, scrolling the stream of videos, had become another platform for open discussions about women's health. I watched one, a pounding beat as TikTok user @that.c00chie.girl announces: '*Here's your daily coochie exercise*'.

Add some repeated 'xo' emojis, and we know what to do.

This is the GripTok challenge.

GripTok is a call mainly to women (men are invited too) to clench and release their pelvic floor to the beat of a song playing in the background of a video. The exercise, more commonly known as a Kegel, is often recommended by doctors to women of childbearing age to strengthen their pelvic floor muscles after they've had a baby, as well as post-menopausal women. Now, however, the GripTok trend has caught on among teenagers, with corresponding hashtags racking up over sixty million views, and an offering of a range of feature songs of alternating speeds and difficulty. A plethora of accounts under names like @dailyreminderladies have emerged to encourage users – some as young as fourteen – to practise their daily reps.

Watching the girls in full make-up, clenching to lyrics that, on the face of it, put the female experience, or at least, the vagina, front and centre, the practice of Kegels seems to have evolved far beyond its modest origins. The technique was developed in the late 1940s by Dr Arnold H. Kegel, an American gynaecologist, as a nonsurgical way to prevent women from leaking urine, a condition known as urinary incontinence. Kegel considered vaginal childbirth to be the cause of decreased pelvic floor muscle strength and believed that while surgery might be effective in ensuring the structure was in place, a further intervention would be needed to restore the muscles to function. The work of a South African colleague, Van Skolkvik, directed him to exercise as the answer. Van

Skolkvik had observed that among a tribe of women in South Africa, midwives performed an exercise, asking new mothers to contract their vaginal muscles around their fingers periodically for several weeks, effectively helping them recover strength in that region.

Kegel set about applying this principle of pelvic muscle exercise in his clinical practice in Los Angeles. In a 1948 paper, he eventually published the results of eighteen years of research recommending that physicians help women locate and strengthen their pelvic floors by placing a finger inside the vagina and contracting the muscles in that area. On applying the technique, however, Dr Kegel's research notes revealed the difficulty many of his patients had in doing Kegels correctly. 'Unless given an opportunity to repeat their efforts under visual control, thereby noting any progress they may make, patients are apt to become discouraged.'

Dr Kegel went on to develop a device called the perineometer, the invention for which he is now known. This device consists of a long tube filled with air which slides inside the vagina. The end of the tube that sticks out of the vagina is sealed and connected to a dial. Squeeze the tube and the dial registers the change in pressure, showing its user whether they're performing the exercise correctly and also allowing them to measure their progress by logging the numbers.

The popularity of Kegel's exercises has fluctuated like the pressure on a perineometer since their introduction, with scientists, physiotherapists and lay sources recommending them for an equally shifting range of symptoms. The advocates spearheading the resurgence of the technique online ascribe benefits that far surpass preventing urinary or even bowel incontinence. The exercises also, various accounts enthuse, 'improve core strength and stability, posture and spinal align-ment' and, most importantly, 'sexual pleasure'. It's remarkable that decades later, the GripTok challenge encourages women to do exactly the same thing. Though this time, less for so-called medical benefits and more for 'empowerment', 'well-ness' and in the name of 'tightness'.

Of the numerous benefits to pelvic floor exercises advocated online, sexual pleasure takes the spotlight. This is also witnessed in the host of so-called 'sextech' purporting to tackle the pelvic region. From the Lioness biofeedback vibrator that tracks pelvic contractions during arousal, to Fitbit-like smart Kegel exercis-ers like Elvie's Trainer (stocked by none other than Goop), to the Ohnut wearable ring to help prevent deep penetration, pelvic health has become synonymous with sexual wellbeing.

Kegel exercises may improve sexual pleasure for women by cultivating stronger muscle which might contract more easily, spurring along the involuntary contraction of the pelvic floor muscles that occur during orgasm and because this exercise promotes blood flow to the pelvic area, increasing sensitivity, although this isn't clear. The sense of control Kegels give can also have a positive psychological impact on women that might enhance sexual pleasure. Whatever the reason, however, it has nothing to do with the 'tightness' that pervades product descriptions of smart Kegel trainer brands. These descriptions reveal how claims that Kegels are 'good for sex' are often less about women's sexual pleasure and more about a coveted aesthetic of vaginal tightness. Yet again, the messages being spread in a spirit of openness, in this case around pelvic floor issues, come dangerously close to that Goop-scented reduction of women's health to a sanitised apology for female biology that must, at all costs, remain 'sexy'.

The wellness empire has formed around a shift that could have been empowering for many women. Despite its wayward direction, it still is for some. Personally, it has allowed me to find solidarity over issues that I was never able to vocalise in the doctor's consultation room. That need for validation and real solutions, however, has been co-opted by an industry that has preyed on a demand, without interrogating where it derives from. It sells us often unfounded 'solutions' to problems that have emerged from age-old sexist thinking about women and their bodies.

As we look to wellness to meet our needs, as in medicine, it is important that we continue to interrogate the messaging about our bodies and our worth, and it is important not to allow this commodified sector to detract from the pressure on medicine itself to cater for women's health and not their sex appeal.

How medicine has let us down

As a child, I had a cousin whose mum had what she called a 'sinking uterus'; a child's interpretation of uterine prolapse. That seemed to me like a terrible precarity to live with, and my childish appetite for the absurd had me sneaking a glance into my aunt's bedroom every time I went to visit them, just to make sure she was still lying down, hadn't stood up in some deluded bout of confidence unleashing her innards. I'd always find her in bed, long scraggly hair just like her daughter's tangled on the pillow. Deserted. And each time I wondered how long it would be until someone saved her.

When I talked to my own mum about our relative with the surreal condition, she told me that she was depressed. Depressed because she was unwell. This was one of my first encounters with the ways in which women's problems can multiply as they carry the stigma and pain of their neglected medical conditions.

There are so many factors that could have kept my aunt in bed. It may have been the physical pain preventing her from moving, embarrassment at possible incontinence, fear at the emerging bulge protruding from her vagina, or it may have been a sense of failure or frustration with the fact that she was unable to do the things she wanted to do – work, be a mother, have relationships, have sex. One thing is certain – her condition affected her in ways that required more than a couple of Kegels or a jade egg to solve.

Even away from the dazzling internet sphere, the promise of 'wellness' – from Kegels, eggs or fragrances – is unavoidable. Doctors and women alike continue to turn to the power of the clench to treat conditions far more severe than urinary incontinence. In her 2020 book *Kegels Are Not Going to Fix This*,[3] neuroscientist Dr Georgeann Sack takes issue with the tendency of friends and doctors to suggest Kegels when she told them about her difficulty trying to find treatment for her uterine prolapse.

Many women experience prolapse post-childbirth. In 10–15% of vaginal deliveries, in fact. The organs within a woman's pelvis (uterus, bladder and rectum) are normally held in place by ligaments and muscles known as the pelvic floor. These muscles come under strain during pregnancy and childbirth, which can lead to stress incontinence – leaking urine when coughing, sneezing or straining and faecal incontinence. It can also lead to pelvic organ prolapse, whereby the pelvic organs bulge from their natural position into the vagina.

Uterine prolapse occurs when the woman's uterus falls down the vaginal canal. It is most common among women who have given birth. The attachment of the muscles to the side walls tears, weakening their ability to support the uterus. And most women won't even know there's a problem until the muscles weaken further with age and are no longer able to hold the organs in place. The condition comes with a host of side effects. As Sack describes in her book: 'I could not pee or poop normally. I leaked urine. Sex hurt. I had a bulge of tissue protruding from my body that created daily discomfort.' As doctors continued to dismiss her problem, Sack had only her intuition to go by, which told her that the damage sustained during childbirth was serious and went deeper than the vaginal tears that had been stitched up after delivery. It took seven years before she discovered that she was experiencing uterine prolapse. 'I was broken,' she writes, 'and Kegels were not going to fix it.'

'*I was broken.*'

It's a sentiment that echoes through the studies on women's experience of uterine prolapse. It's a sentiment that is internalised when women scour social media for the latest trend that will 'fix' them or make them better.

The idea of the female body as defective or deficient (and therefore the female too) is not new, of course. It was scrawled onto Egyptian papyruses, etched into medieval woodcuts – even the Bible instructs that prolapse is a sign a wife has been unfaithful.[4] These diagnoses led to what were considered to be the appropriate treatments: fumigating the lower abdomen with herbs, as we have seen; tying women upside-down to a ladder and shaking it; or a hot poker to taunt the unruly uterus, menacing it back into place.[5] We've already encountered the historical idea that women's reproductive systems are somehow dirty. Here, we see how this belief was associated with women as defective and temperamental, and that these qualities came to describe not just the body but the woman too. Like I said, vaginal steaming isn't new.

This dismissive cultural attitude exists today in the idea that uterine prolapse is just an inevitable consequence of childbirth or of being a woman. This attitude allows doctors to side-step giving the condition serious medical attention. In an article in the *Washington Post*, Carmel Price, a sociology professor at Michigan University, like Sack, describes the dismissive attitude of doctors towards her condition even in the process of arranging surgery: 'My ob-gyn said, "Oh, your body just changes after having a baby" and it's just life . . .' Dr Price, 38, has since made prolapse the focus of her sociological research. She describes how her doctor made surgery seem elective, not strictly necessary, pointing out, 'My dad has had shoulder surgery and I never heard the term quality of life, like if he's just willing to stop playing golf then his shoulder is not a problem.'

We have here a double standard that deems non-life-threatening medical problems in women minor quality of life issues, while in men they merit serious medical intervention. This medical dismissiveness towards their problems means that rather than pointing to inadequate medical support, women tend to blame themselves for their deteriorating conditions. In a 2019 study[6] that interviewed women undergoing medical treatment for prolapse in the UK, the subjects attributed their condition to a range of factors, including higher number of pregnancies, a lack of general exercise throughout life, hormonal imbalances, a persistent cough and ageing. These risk factors were coupled with the idea that their own lifestyle choices – and so only they themselves – were to blame. Those who were most accepting of prolapse considered it to be an inevitable and irreversible part of ageing. They seemed resigned to the symptoms because they believed nothing could be done to mitigate them, and they blamed their defective lifestyles and failing bodies for their onset and decline.

This medical neglect, this displacement of blame onto women rather than healthcare, has rendered these conditions invisible in a way that their counterparts – torn ligaments in shoulders, knees or hips – are not. This often manifests in misguided advice given to women by their doctors. An insistence on Kegels, in the cases where prolapse is taken seriously, seems strange, coming from medical professionals who should know that there has been no convincing research showing that these will help. In so-called 'conservative' cases of prolapse, where the muscle has only weakened, there is some evidence that regular Kegels will help restore the muscle and relieve some of the side effects like urinary incontinence. However, none of the problems with perseverance has gone away since Kegel invented them, and these exercises take a hefty commitment (about twenty repetitions three times a day) for small improvements of around 17% compared to no treatment. In the cases where pelvic floor muscle weakness results from torn muscle, exercise will do nothing to repair them and will require surgery or an alternative like a pessary, an internal support device that a woman can insert to hold the uterus in place.

Yet somehow, the idea of sending women with prolapse home to do their exercises has persisted as an appealing solution in medical practice. I asked John DeLancey, Professor of

Gynaecology at the University of Michigan, who pioneered the use of MRI scans and biomechanical analysis to diagnose pelvic floor damage, why he thought the condition wasn't being correctly treated. He told me that from his clinical experience, the problem wasn't a lack of clinical options but of communication.

'There is no language around prolapse,' Professor DeLancey told me from his home study. Unlike incontinence which has a word and recognisable symptoms, 'with prolapse, I often see people struggling to say what's bothering them'. He recalled an investigation his department attempted in the early 2000s, where they asked women with prolapse or incontinence who they would feel comfortable disclosing their symptoms to. Their findings showed that information tends to spread by word of mouth rather than via books or experts – through neighbourhoods, communities and families. Doctors were definitely not the first port of call. This is another example of how the vacuum left by a lack of medical attention to women's specific health problems can be filled; just as in wellness, perhaps this can point us to new, innovative ways to meet that need, but it can also breed misinformation and detract from pressure on the medical system itself to step up.

Professor DeLancey's sense that patients' discussions with doctors about prolapse are stunted is echoed in surveys that have been conducted. The 2019 UK study showed how patients' inability to discuss their symptoms of prolapse meant that health professionals' own preferences tended to shape treatment. Consultants who doubted the effectiveness of physiotherapy presented surgery more favourably than alternatives like the pessary, suggesting to women that they try physiotherapy, but that they'd still need surgery eventually. Others pushed for the physiotherapy that was becoming a more popular course of treatment at the time. And many women reported receiving little or no choice in their treatment decisions, the end result often inconsistent with their preferences and needs.

Studies such as these on the experiences of women in their treatment for prolapse are rare. Nonetheless, they already help to elucidate the issue around communication noted by Professor DeLancey. They show, for example, that although patients' silence on their symptoms might be at play, what is more significant is that doctors are dominating the conversation.

Gynos exist in silos – that is, there is here a problem of practitioners being unable to think beyond the narrow limitations of what has become regular practice. Surgeons justify their choice of operations in papers claiming these to be scientifically preferable, when they are determined by the culture not just of their field but of their specific hospital. As these doctors forge ahead implementing what to them is just scientific, neutral, 'evidence-based medicine', they are unable to mould their approach to the needs of their patients.

You can see how a doctor with what they believe to be an authoritative stance on the issue might not invite a patient to express their preferences. Perhaps doctors have siloed themselves from their patients, and thereby aren't facilitating an environment that makes women comfortable to discuss their problems. Women do find the words to talk about their pelvic floor problems – they find ways to communicate them to friends and family. They just don't feel able to do so in a consultation room. Perhaps the problem isn't that patients aren't talking but that medicine isn't listening, that it hasn't found a way to engage its patients in meaningful conversation.

If gynaecologists have noticed a silence among patients on their symptoms of prolapse, the responsibility has to fall to the medical profession that holds the expertise in the subject area to cultivate discussion. The watershed moment in women's health relies on medicine responding to women's specific needs and opening up new medical frontiers. If it doesn't, women are left wide open to suggestions of alternative methods – methods that go hand in hand with the commodification of harmful practices like vaginal steaming, at the cost of reinforcing and further internalising sexist ideas about them and their bodies. So, medicine must learn to *listen*.

But it's not quite that simple. According to Dr Sinéad Dufour, long-practising pelvic health physiotherapist and Assistant Clinical Professor in the Faculty of Health Science at McMaster University, Canada, in order to do this, medicine must learn how to ask the right questions. Dr Dufour also works as Assistant Instructor at Pelvic Health Solutions. This evidence-based teaching company was founded, in 2010, in Ontario, to educate healthcare professionals about pelvic health and restoring pelvic health through physiotherapy. Dr Dufour and her colleagues attend various hospitals and advise staff predominantly on the questions they need to ask to help patients identify symptoms. Using a straightforward survey, patients can identify risk factors for prolapse or incontinence, asking women whether they experience symptoms like frequent urination or leakage, as well as abdominal or genital pain, and to what degree, using a sliding scale. This avoids some of the problems around women feeling reluctant to report symptoms or a tendency to minimise symptoms so that they go undiagnosed. This form, Dr Dufour asserts, could easily be incorporated into the regular appointment women have for cervical screenings. This, along with standard pelvic floor assessments, could go a long way in providing often very straightforward solutions to life-inhibiting problems, and in many cases prevent them from escalating.

As with many gynaecological issues, pelvic health problems are common, and they even arise at predictable points in a woman's lifespan. And as with many gynaecological issues, one effective solution is to simply (and admittedly a little unsexily) add some admin to the process. It seems inexcusable not to incorporate something as straightforward as an appropriately timed conversation into regular care when this can make all the difference.

Pelvic health physiotherapists are leading the charge on initiating the discussions that will encourage women to seek help for their pelvic floor problems. Many have turned to social media platforms, especially Instagram, to inform women that conditions like incontinence are common but not normal, and that simple solutions are available. Social media, just like any other form of media, can be used to inform as well as misinform. It's not all GripTok. Very informative accounts include 'embodywellnesspt', 'drsarahduvall', 'krystyna_holland' and 'dr.sinead' herself. Through these profiles, physiotherapists provide information on reducing pain and other symptoms – as Dr Dufour put it, 'shouting from the hilltops', providing essential information until 'pelvic floor assessment has become a regular component of primary healthcare'. I think about how much conversations like these, surveys like these, could have helped my aunt. How many years of suffering – psychological and physical – she could have avoided if the right questions had been asked, if she had been heard.

While social media accounts tend to focus predominantly on pregnant and postpartum women with pelvic floor disorders, there has yet to be a similar outreach effort for ageing women. Dr Sack argues that protocols to assess pelvic health, built into important moments in routine healthcare, need to be extended to older women. The risk of pelvic health issues is highest for women over sixty-five, and so these women in particular need to be assessed for pelvic floor disorders at least once every few years post-menopause. Every assisted living facility should also include pelvic floor disorder assessment via questionnaires and referral to urogynaecologists or physical therapists, as needed.

'It can be a scary thing to lose control of bladder or bowels or to suddenly have a bulge sticking out of your vagina,' Dr Sack commented. 'Many ageing women in particular are embarrassed to talk about these problems with doctors.' It falls to the doctor to ensure these discussions are held. 'If your doctor doesn't list these symptoms women may not think to mention them.' You develop a patient-centric language by asking the right questions and listening to the answers.

Listening to women, it turns out, is exactly what the medical field has been missing out on. This emphasis on asking the right questions, for example, aligns with women's own suggestions for improvements to the treatment of uterine prolapse. In the 2019 UK study, women emphasised the importance of prevention education before symptoms started to appear. They suggested emphasising the importance of pelvic floor exercises in postnatal checks for example and called for drop-in clinics to provide opportunities to discuss symptoms and identify any problems earlier on. To achieve timely diagnosis and intervention, women also called for greater awareness and training for GPs on early identification of prolapse symptoms and available treatment options. GPs need to be more proactive, they said. The fact that the assessment of patients aligns with that of the most forward-thinking researchers in the field suggests that there is a wealth of knowledge, latent among patients, that should not be wasted as the field flows to new terrain.

Once they start these discussions with their patients, doctors may find that the best treatment may not align with what they perceive to be cutting-edge science. Once again, the best science may not be sexy. Surgery, for example, though generally effective,* is not without risks. To some, a non-surgical intervention, such as a pessary, may be preferable. Pessaries may cause discharge and have to be removed prior to sex, but there are no real risks involved, and they allow women to move about freely and do the kind of heavy lifting that would not be possible post-surgery. Women can weigh up their options with regards to their needs and lifestyles, if informed.

In the UK study that asked women about their treatment, physiotherapy-based interventions emerged as very helpful in helping them regain control over their symptoms and life. Neither patients, GPs nor consultants sufficiently incorporated this option into treatment, perhaps because as we have seen in the case of torn muscles, these techniques don't provide a 'cure' for the disease. Yet physiotherapy nonetheless proved helpful to women because it gave them a sense of control in the form of techniques that they felt helped them manage their symptoms. They talked for example about being able to do the things they had been unable to do due to the side effects of incontinence, like sneeze or cough while out walking, getting out and going further without needing the toilet. Studies of

* Professor DeLancey performed a study at his Michigan clinic showing that seven years after surgery, 90% of people were satisfied with the results.

the experiences of women will remind doctors that this sense of agency can be as important as physical improvement. And at the very least, an increased sense of agency, an increased level of control over symptoms and quality of life, are the very things that will prevent women – often in desperation for an option, any option – from turning to the sometimes harmful methods suggested by wellbeing organisations.

If there is some benefit to Kegel exercises for prolapse, they should be incorporated into women's lives in a way that maximises the latter's sense of agency and control. Once again, doctors need to listen and treatment should respond to women's indicated needs, not be imposed. In this way, the GripTok trend might actually be of some help in that it helps girls identify their pelvic muscles early on, allowing them to identify and express any problems later down the line.

Janis Miller, an obstetrics and gynaecology professor and pelvic floor researcher at the University of Michigan, suggests it would be beneficial to teach girls to squeeze pelvic floor muscles when they cough or sneeze and after using the bathroom. 'If girls and adolescents could just . . . be brought aware of this muscle, instead of this being a secret, hidden thing, and start using it, then we wouldn't need to set aside time every day to do Kegel exercises.'

Dr Sack also has a recommendation – the 'modern Kegel'. This version of the exercise integrates the Kegel with breathing which allows you to contract the pelvic floor with support from the diaphragm. Dr Sack says she prefers this type of Kegel because it is easy to incorporate into exercise, especially yoga and Pilates, making it easier for women to integrate it into their daily lives without setting aside time to Kegel each day.

It seems apt that the connection between breathing and Kegels is a dimension that has been overlooked – the relationship between the pelvic floor and that continuous motion that continues across a life. It is once again a symptom of the siloed thinking that fails to listen and respond to women's needs across a life course.

The relationship to breathing was elucidated by an equally overlooked early female pioneer of the technique. The pelvic floor exercises named after Arnold Kegel first entered modern medicine in 1936, in a paper by the dancer-turned-physiotherapist Margaret Morris who had developed the technique after realising that her dancers' health and posture improved with breathing techniques. In 1930, she had co-authored the St Thomas' Hospital paper, 'Maternity and Post-Operative Exercises', which explained the importance of breathing and posture before, during and after labour. In her 1936 paper, Morris described tensing and relaxing the pelvic floor muscle as a preventative treatment for urinary and faecal incontinence, introducing pelvic floor exercise to the British physiotherapy profession – before Kegel established this as a widespread practice in the US.

Recovering Morris's legacy reminds us of the importance of interdisciplinarity, but also importantly female practitioners in the field who are more attune to women's lived experience. The modern Kegel caters to the modern woman by refusing to rely solely on motivational perineometers or any of the digitised variants. The new approach makes Kegels more sustainable and, importantly, doesn't ask women to hide away in their homes, concealing and internalising their struggle as they sweat away in silence. Kegels can be integrated, stigma-free, into the active lifestyles of modern women.

There is much to be optimistic about in the field of pelvic floor disorders. With scientific advances increasingly allowing surgeons to identify the root cause of prolapse, more direct and effective surgeries are imminent. Also promising is that the field is growing. In the US, the National Institutes of Health (NIH) opened applications specifically on pelvic floor disorders in 1999. As a result, the number of published research papers on pelvic floor disorders has steadily increased over the last twenty years. As of 2011, Female Pelvic Medicine and Reconstructive Surgery is an accredited subspecialty with fellowships, exams and certification – the first oral certifying exam in 2015. This all means that there is a growing number of doctors with several years of additional training in the diagnosis and treatment of pelvic floor disorders specifically.

Most encouraging, however, are the calls for protocols to ensure that there is ongoing discussion around women's pelvic floor health allowing preventative care. In the UK, the Royal College of Obstetricians and Gynaecologists (RCOG) have made important recommendations in their bid for better, more integrated healthcare for women. In their 2019 report, RCOG called for pre-and postnatal appointments to have a stronger emphasis on pelvic floor exercises and information about the importance of a healthy pelvic floor. These should also, they write, be discussed at ongoing interactions with the health service, such as at the NHS Health Check or at cervical cancer screening appointments, regardless of whether a woman has been pregnant or given birth. They also highlight the need for lifestyle advice, and say that at all interactions with the NHS, women should be encouraged to make healthy lifestyle choices – such as weight management, avoiding heavy lifting and not smoking – that will reduce the risk of getting prolapse or could stop mild symptoms from getting worse. These measures are all geared towards ongoing, sustained dialogue between women and healthcare professionals.

As I think about this progress, the image of my aunt returns to me, the tangle of her hair on the pillow reminding me of the true tragedy of her situation – that the solutions to her problems weren't necessarily complicated, but rather reflected a general neglect of women's medical-related issues. The tools that would have helped her were, in fact, available: all they required was conversation. My aunt's condition might also have been preventable had there been more regular checks and advice after she gave birth to my cousin. Had she been made to feel that her body and her quality of life mattered. But she didn't feel at that time that she mattered so she lay in bed while her husband played video games downstairs and while my cousin picked up the household slack. My aunt was made to feel that she wasn't worth helping and my cousin, the next generation, received these self-same messages about self-sacrifice the longer she was expected to quietly run a household instead of playing and learning and exploring as I was lucky enough to be able to do.

Years later, after we'd moved away and lost touch, my mum and I bumped into my cousin and my aunt – who now stood firmly upright, on her own two feet. She had left her husband, she told us, had surgery, moved away and had sent my cousin to a school that challenged her. 'My daughter is top of her class,' she wanted us to know. My cousin was happy and I could tell she knew how much she was capable of. And it reassured me that she would always know that she was worthy of getting the help she needed, because her mother had done it and it had changed both of their lives. This is what pelvic floor health is about. Not about marketised sexiness, but giving women the ability to thrive in this society. For generations to come.

Rethinking our bodies

A boyfriend once asked me, quite genuinely I think, why I spent so much time thinking about bodies in general and my own body in particular. To him, he said, a body was just an 'eating and fucking machine'. The delivery was lacking in subtlety, and perhaps even empathy, but I don't think that was his intention. In a way, he had put his finger on the problem. Women do spend a lot of time thinking about their bodies. Not through any fault of our own, but instead, simply by existing in a culture that perpetually confronts us with the limitations of our bodies, while at the same time telling us that our bodies define us, give us value as sexualised objects and baby-makers.

We spend time wondering about undiagnosed and untreated issues within our bodies. We are ashamed to go and get the help we need to treat our bodies. We worry that our bodies have failed and try to understand how our bodies should look and be. The wellness industry mirrors this failure back at us under the guise of a celebration of femininity. This sleight of hand is familiar – perhaps that's why we're drawn to it. Maybe that familiarity explains why we're prepared to settle for a glimmer of acknowledgement. We're used to the darkness of isolation, after all.

I was so excited when I discovered in my twenties that there were open conversations happening online, that there were products marketed to helping me to understand my body, and then perhaps, even, stop thinking about my body at last. Yet in trying to claim some agency over our physical being, women are tragically subjected to yet more sexism, further harmful myths that prize a specific version of sexiness and femininity over health. Medicine needs to take responsibility for women's gynaecology, because, unlike companies like Goop, it has the resources it needs to tackle this lack of understanding – the research tools, the scientists brimming with curiosity, the carers who want to help – it just needs to apply these in new ways, to new problems. It is the state of the field of gynaecology that has women frantically hitting refresh on the page for a sold-out c.$66 jade egg. Once medicine takes the leap to reconsider what it thought it knew, it will discover that, as much as 'bad' feminism, as in, feminism disguising patriarchal messages, leads to substandard pseudo-scientific interventions and a lazy form of practising medicine, good feminism leads to good science too.

And good science means there won't be any room left for wellness companies that capitalise on silence. And so, we'll unplug the gaps left in gynaecology and obstetrics, currently blocked by jade eggs, breaking through with the relevant information needed to heal, not harm, female bodies.

Chapter 4

Sexology

At eighteen, I decided it was high time I had sex. I invited my boyfriend over. He brought condoms (we both knew that was the beginning and the end of his responsibility where child-bearing was concerned) and we assumed our positions on the bed. We knew what to do. I lay under him, he mounted me. Just like the animals on the Discovery Channel. He thrusted enthusiastically and I tried to stop the pain from registering on my face. He came. And we knew it was done. That was the Law of the Kingdom.

The ease with which I slipped into submission at eighteen, the fact that I knew my role without being told, bears uncanny resemblance to the way in which a woman in a doctor's office knows just to oblige, to silence herself, to submit to authority. That resemblance is no coincidence. We have already seen how sexiness is mobilised in science and the medicine of women's health to champion male-centric research avenues and to limit the care available to women in reproductive health.

Sex is a powerful word that dazzles and blinds people. Sexiness in these cases is anything but intimate, but it does describe a relationship. The sex that sells is a version of sex we have all been raised to revere – one in which a man is the penetrator, the arbiter of power, the woman submissive, the passive receptacle. This relationship exists in science as much as it does in our subconscious as we enter into sex; it is a relationship that pervades a patriarchal society in which women are continually told to submit. It should come as no surprise then that it also exists in the science of sex itself.

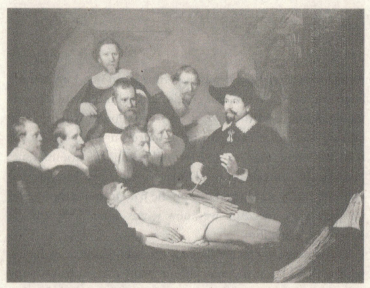

The Anatomy Lesson of Dr Nicolaes Tulp, painted in 1632 by Rembrandt van Rijn. The scene shows a group of Amsterdam surgeons observing how a naked body is being dissected by their teacher. The body belongs to a petty thief, Adriaan Adriaanszoon, who was hanged for his minor crimes.[1]

When I think about the relationship between scientist or clinician and patient, of what it's been, and of how it feels to me, a particular image from my Dutch cultural heritage haunts me. Rembrandt van Rijn's *The Anatomy Lesson of Dr Nicolaes Tulp*, painted in 1632, depicts a group of Amsterdam surgeons, all bearded and dressed in black, hovering over a naked body being dissected. The body is vulnerable, exposed to the brazenly inquisitive mob. I spent a lot of time staring at the painting in the Mauritshuis in The Hague. I found it again, later, in the book *The Rings of Saturn*, by writer and academic W. G. Sebald, which helped explain its resonance. The picture, Sebald writes, is dominated by the absent presence of the identity of the corpse being dissected. The body belongs to 'Adriaan Adriaanszoon alias Aris Kindt, a petty thief of that city who had been hanged for his misdemeanours an hour or so earlier'[2] but that no longer matters. It no longer matters who this man was or is by the time his body reaches the dissection table. While the other men – upper-class, educated – loom over him, study every detail of his body in meticulous detail, his identity is deemed irrelevant in this highly scientific context. I think that the image of Enlightenment science haunted me because it was suffused with a power dynamic I intuitively recognised. The image sent shivers down my spine because it confronted me with a powerlessness at the hands of medical professionals that felt familiar to me. I recognised the medical procedures that are also rituals reinforcing social assumptions about whose bodies are valued. All this in a system that turns individuals to anonymous flesh under the guise of scientific neutrality. Operating threatres aren't always the site of this performance, sometimes it is the consultation room, or the laboratory, but the dynamic in which the body under inspection surrenders to the 'all-knowing' eye of the professional is at the foundation of our medical system. This is a science that would rather know than be curious, because any challenge to its absolute authority threatens to expose the subjugation that makes knowing possible. This is a science that has succumbed to the uncouth, dare I say almost erotic, desire to gaze over debilitated flesh, flesh that scientists claim to know better than it knew itself.

The model of the knowing scientist or doctor versus ignorant body of the patient persists today. It is a dynamic we're groomed into in our daily lives – the expert versus the lay person. It's also a dynamic that we fall into too easily in the bedroom. It is a relationship in which those in power – often the men – do all the penetrating. It is a relationship that consolidates male power, male desire and male pleasure. Perhaps this centrality of male desire to our social world explains why, where science and sex meet explicitly, in the field of sexology, scientists have struggled to respond to research that has challenged this powerful, power-ridden status quo. Research that threatened male sovereignty over pleasure, showing that women orgasm, that women have sexual thoughts, that women know their desires just as men do, that women even ejaculate like men.

In sexology, the penetrative gaze of science conspires with the penetrations of penises to limit any investigation to consolidating a status quo. Findings showing the active role of women in sexual intercourse threaten to take the penis off its pedestal, after all, and the cultural implications of this shift are huge. They challenge male supremacy. They are subversive. They provide new insights into pleasure, a better scientific understanding of sexual health, but also, for medicine as a whole, might help us undo the missionary position medicine maintains across its fields of inquiry, to rethink not only how it sees women but also how it learns about bodies in general.

Female ejaculation – debunking myths

If male penetration is the status quo, if a man inseminating a woman is how we have come to understand sex and science and our roles within them, then for women there is no better scientific fuel for resistance than the phenomenon of female ejaculation. The conceptually subversive power of the image of an ejaculating female body has posed a challenge to sexologists since the inception of the field, undoing everything they thought they knew about male and female bodies at a time when they were still developing their scientific scaffolding. Their response was a classic one we'll see repeatedly when scientists have been confronted with findings that challenge their gendered assumptions: dismissal and denial, at the cost of women's credibility and their sense of agency over their own bodies. But let me be clear: female ejaculation is real. It has been reported, recorded. It has even been filmed.

The field of sexology emerged in the 1960s, with a series of taboo-breaking studies into human sexuality. The US obstetrician and gynaecologist William Masters and his research assistant and later co-researcher Virginia Johnson have been credited as its pioneers. Pioneers of sexology – that is quite a claim to fame. Their research into human sexual response and the diagnosis and treatment of sexual disorders and dysfunctions dispelled many long-standing misconceptions about women as asexual. Their findings, particularly on the nature of female sexual arousal (for example, describing the mechanisms of vaginal lubrication and debunking the earlier widely held notion that this originated from the cervix) and orgasm (proving, among other things, that some women were capable of having multiple orgasms), opened up the space to investigate female orgasm as on a par with male ejaculation. Yet while the pair are often discussed in the context of the sexual liberation movement, as veritable drivers alongside the likes of leading feminist Germaine Greer, their research reflected, often implicitly, many of the traditional assumptions about male dominance we have seen. In doing so, they missed opportunities to understand the female sexual response. Their failure to understand female ejaculation, still not fully understood today, in particular, reveals the limits of their emancipation and, in doing so, they set the tone in the field for the decades to come.

As in obstetrics and gynaecology, where a very narrow understanding of female sexuality obliterated issues like prolapse, as we have seen, or a more holistic approach to gynaecology from the scientific purview, in sexology, too, ideas about how women are behaving and how they are supposed to behave have blinded scientists. They didn't believe what women's bodies were telling them, or what women were telling them about their bodies because they were looking through a tightly framed ideological lens that ignored and erased any evidence that would expand their view.

Today, sexology is an expanding and evolving field, its practitioners increasingly diverse, along with their methods. But, as with the rest of medicine, it remains entrenched in scientific approaches that have formed around narrowly framed questions. The impact of LGBTQIA+ movements in particular has shifted and transformed research models and cultural thinking about the study of sexuality. As in gynaecology and obstetrics, scholars and practitioners have begun to challenge the disease prevention model that still dominates in the field. While behavioural research like that of Masters and Johnson is needed to help prevent social problems or tackle disease, some argue that this preventive approach has also meant that sexology research and its questions are generally geared towards motivating behavioural change, while conceptualising sexuality in a negative or problematic context, according to prevailing cultural-determined gender biases. There is a growing call for work that looks at the complex relations between social movements, community structure, personal identity and sexual practices, and also at the biological and social interactions that impact sexual life.

Biological factors such as hormonal influences and genetics should be studied in a social and cultural context that reflects the complexity of human sexuality. In the case of the sexuality of women, this might include investigations into the interactions of biological factors, such as hormones, and psychological factors, such as power dynamics or tensions in negotiating sexual interactions, along with the potential effects of stress or feelings about pregnancy on women's sexuality. For women in same-sex relationships, questions might include what the effects of new family structures, a growing 'out-culture' or a social acceptance or rejection of same-sex partnerships might be on sexual behaviour or the formation of new sexual scripts. Sexology research has done a lot to break down barriers and tackle taboos, but being a part of patriarchal culture, like all other fields of medicine, it has also reinforced existing, often sexist, misconceptions.

In its early days, the social progressiveness of sexology was assumed, and much of its research was even adopted by the feminist movement. But the social assumptions guiding the research itself remained oblique. In their early 1966 laboratory research, Masters and Johnson were supposed to be investigating what happened to men and women as they responded to effective sexual stimulation. Yet when some of their female research participants reported a sensation of ejaculating fluid during orgasm, the pair dismissed these observations as insignificant. Their rationale – that they believed that women's reports had been misinterpreted by male researchers.

> During the first stage of subjective progression in orgasm, the sensation of intense clitoral-pelvic awareness has been described by a number of women as occurring concomitantly with a sense of bearing down or expelling. Often a feeling of receptive opening was expressed. This last sensation was reported only by parous study subjects, a small number of whom expressed some concept of having an actual fluid emission or of expending in some concrete fashion. Previous male interpretation of these subjective reports may have resulted in the erroneous but widespread concept that female ejaculation is an integral part of female orgasmic expression.[3]

Reading this now, it seems ironic that these researchers who clung to a conceptual framework that reinforced a male-dominated sexual 'norm' dismissed women's own experiences as the consequences of that very same overrepresented male perspective. Perhaps, as they wrote, female ejaculation isn't integral to every woman's sexual experience, but is that a reason to dismiss it as a scientific question worth investigating altogether?

Had Masters and Johnson done some historical research to complement their science, they would have found that reports of female ejaculation were anything but new and had, indeed, been recorded for centuries across different societies. In a 2010 article, the urologist Dr Joanna Korda and her colleagues showed how ancient Eastern and Western texts alike already differentiated between vaginal lubrication during sex and the rarer external ejaculation of sexual fluids. In ancient India, for example, the *Kama Sutra*, which dates to 200–400 A.D., mentions 'female semen' that 'falls continually'. In the West, even Aristotle had something to say about female discharge during sexual intercourse, which he pointed out, 'far exceeds' the seminal emission of the man. In the seventeenth century, Dutch anatomist Regnier de Graaf described the fluid once again, also linking it to an erogenous zone inside the vagina that resembled the male prostate.

Masters and Johnson didn't find evidence that would support the women's reports because they didn't look for it. This methodological choice reverberates through the field and its response to female ejaculation, and moreover, in its response to self-reporting by females in general. It is a choice to value a certain kind of observed, but directed, 'scientific' evidence over the anecdotal, 'unscientific' evidence provided by women about their own bodies. The assumption underlying this epistemological distinction is that sex revolves around the male experience, expressed as a performance of male pleasure. We see once again that patriarchal science – seen repeatedly in art, literature and research – a science that erases its guiding assumptions to reaffirm its power structures in the form of an 'objective' scientific method. But that is guided by assumptions about whose perspective matters: that of the scientist over the patient and of the man over the woman.

Masters and Johnson's rejection of female ejaculation begins to reveal that the scientific refusal to study women's bodies on their own terms is coupled with a general rejection of women's reported experiences in favour of existing scientific ideas. In sexology, the female perspective is not regarded as scientific. Their words, like their physiological responses, are discarded as anomalies when they don't prop up the man-is-dominant stereotype.

Given that the methods in sexology were designed to measure a desire that was presumed to be exclusive to men, it's fascinating to read how their tools, when applied to women, failed them.

In one study conducted in 2004 by Meredith Chivers and colleagues in Ontario, Canada,[4] researchers measured the physiological arousal of men and women using a measuring device called a 'plethysmograph'. This was attached to participants' respective genitalia to measure their physiological response to a range of videos of men, women and animals who were just naked or also having sex. The researchers found a contrast between men and women in their findings that was difficult to explain. While they measured genital arousal in men only in the cases where they reported to be aroused, the women responded with genital arousal to every clip. The women showed little of what the researchers called 'category specificity' compared to men according to these physiological measures. But what is interesting to me is not so much the discrepancy between men and women, but that between the types of results collected for women. In addition to the physiological data, the researchers collected 'subjective' reports of arousal. These results showed that while women were physically aroused by the whole range of videos, they would often say that they weren't. This 'non-concordance' between their genital arousal and their subjective sense of arousal led researchers to conclude that the women were confused.

In their report, this 'non-concordance' is the conclusion of the study. But I agree with the author and academic Katherine Angel, who in her nuanced exploration of female desire, *Tomorrow Sex Will Be Good Again*,[5] argues that this so-called non-concordance could and should have prompted further investigation into the women's responses. Perhaps this discrepancy points not to some kind of inconsistency in women's experience but to the limitations of the scientific tools used to gauge them. The findings could have prompted the researchers to investigate the reasons for their reported arousal or non-arousal. The findings were begging the researchers to look beyond simple physiological markers to develop more evolved measures of women's desire. Instead, the conclusion they drew was one of discordance, and the solution, it was implied, would be to reduce their experience somehow to existing metrics. The plethysmograph had to be right. As Angel states, it was a lie detector, 'a penetrative probe' that was 'believed to access the truth about women's sexuality'. The physiological gauge told the truth of women's words; accounts that deviated revealed the inconsistency of women, not the incompatibility of tools designed to measure their desire by male physiological standards.

Given this history of sexology's dismissal of women's accounts, it now seems less surprising that in the research on female ejaculation, the importance of women's words has been subsumed by the hunt for physiological, existing scientific explanations. While Dr Amy Gilliland's 2009 study,[6] based on women's own accounts, has been one of the most useful and widely cited on female ejaculation to date, similar research on women's subjective experience of ejaculation has not been done since. 'No research has been done in this area for over 20 years,' lamented Dr Gilliland in a 2011 *Scientific American* article,[7] 'and we still do not have an answer satisfying to most sexologists as to what female ejaculate fluid is or where it is manufactured.'

I spoke to Dr Gilliland in 2021, over Zoom. Red hair blazing, she spoke to me from a jam-packed study, excited, it seemed, to revisit a subject she'd relegated to her archives. The obstacles to research, she told me, remain the same as when she began her study and tried to get it published in 2004. The article was rejected by the journal *Sex Research* after it was reviewed by a urologist who opined that because it wasn't yet known where the fluid expelled in female ejaculation came from, it wouldn't be scientifically valid to publish the article. Dr Gilliland tried to explain at the time that the aim of the study wasn't to identify the physiological basis of female ejaculation but to describe and understand women's experiences. To no avail. It was easier to focus on measurable biological phenomena, using established scientific methods. Within a scientific methodology that only registers, and so can only try to explain, quantifiable, physiological response, the truth in words, especially divergent truths, don't register.

The scientific method has evolved around the primacy of male experience and authority. Male-dominated science asserts its truths in the form of measured physiological response reflecting the primacy of male experience in sex, at the cost of the unquantifiable, unscientific, unimportant words of women. The tools that scientists have developed to measure their results reflect these hierarchies of knowledge and power. What if we were to develop different metrics? Can we find the tools to investigate new dimensions of sex? What if, once again, we let the watershed of female words guide us to new places? What would we find? What would the science of sex look like? What would sex look like?

Dr Gilliland was eventually able to publish her story by capitalising on the cultural moment that came with what she calls the 'Oprahfication' of American society, a term she uses to describe the impact of African American broadcaster Oprah Winfrey's 1986–2011 daytime syndicated talk show, which remains one of the highest-rated in US history. The show did a lot to normalise women talking about their 'dysfunctional relationships with other people', Dr Gilliland commented, allowing women to feel more open talking about their private lives. This trickled through to the culture of the people running scientific journals, who began to accept studies that took subjective experiences seriously. Dr Gilliland's struggle to get her study published is just another example of the ways in which the cultural moment shapes the conversations we are able to have in and about science. Culture, still dominated by a male perspective, creates the conditions that allow women to speak and be heard about their bodies.

Since the 1980s, women have been filming their own ejaculation in part as evidence of the elusive myth, but also as a challenge to medicine to take women and their bodies seriously. In her 1981 seminal work on the G-spot, American sexologist Beverly Whipple worked with filmmaker Mark Schoen to release a nine-minute video, *Orgasmic Expulsions of Fluid in the Sexually Stimulated Female*. This proved without a doubt that women squirted liquid during sex. Filmed evidence should have made it impossible for anyone, including scientists, to deny that female ejaculation exists, but even the camera is rendered unscientific, it seems, when held by the hands of women. Most scientists responded by protesting that the woman was only expelling urine, that this wasn't, couldn't be, an equivalent to the male ejaculate. Regardless, Whipple set an important precedent as a woman documenting her own body, taking up her own tools to tell the truth of her experience.

Others used the video camera not only to make themselves heard to scientists but also to challenge the scientific scripts that denied them a voice. The pioneering performance philosopher Dr Shannon Bell worked with filmmaker Kath Daymond in 1990 to create *Nice Girls Don't Do It*, the first film on female ejaculation. The film was what Dr Bell calls a '13-minute truth pastiche of knowledge, porn and technical instruction'. While referencing the tropes of pornography with its explicit close-ups, leather and out-of-focus shots, it is filmed in black and white and interposes images with text, leaving blank space for the viewer to (re)interpret the images, to challenge them, to connect them into a different narrative that foregrounds the woman's experience, instead of the man's.

Female ejaculation, in this framing, is appropriately unfamiliar, inviting the viewer to reimagine what sex might look like from the vantage point of a woman and her expressions, physiological or otherwise, of her own desire. Filming female ejaculation outside the context of scientific studies, and beyond the conventions of male-centric porn, challenges the conventional focus on male domination and female subjugation reflected in a focus on penile erection and ejaculation. It also challenges scientists to think about the frameworks they use to understand sexual response. If not in medicine, in what context would women be taken for their word? By contrasting the contexts in which women's bodies and experiences are visible and those where they aren't, Dr Bell urges her viewers to consider why. As long as female experience remains 'unscientific', relegated to the worlds of porn and performance, rather than the laboratory, medicine can continue deferring to its male default. A male perspective continues to dictate the meaning of sex.

Despite women's recordings, scientists have been incredibly innovative in finding new grounds on which to dismiss female ejaculation as a biological process comparable to that of men. Mostly, though, these rejections have drawn on this same distinction between ejaculate and urine, with scientists eager to distil the chemical composition of female ejaculate, to dismiss it as urine. These studies reflect the same conviction, as sex educator Ev'Yan Whitney puts it, that 'scientists know women's bodies better than women know their bodies themselves'.[8] They show how scientific research seems driven by an impulse to counteract, rather than explain, women's reports, to dominate and possess, rather than collaborate and explore. A recipe for bad sex and bad science too.

Over the years, numerous scientists have tried to refute Whipple's findings – to explain them away, find any avenue with which to dispute an overt, physical expression of female pleasure. Some researchers continue to argue that the liquid we now know 40% of women report having produced liberally at least once in their lives is just urine. They are *adamant*. In a 2014 French study, a sample of women were asked to urinate before sex, and then to undertake ultrasound scans to confirm their bladders were empty. They were given a second ultrasound scan after they became aroused, which showed that their bladders had refilled. A third scan once they had ejaculated showed that their bladders had emptied again, suggesting that the liquid ejaculated is at least in part urine.

Nonetheless, almost all studies since the first conducted by Whipple, in the early 1980s, have shown a chemical dissimilarity between urine and female ejaculate. There are, in fact more commonalities with male seminal fluid. Besides microscopic quantities of the chemical constituents of urine, urea and creatine, researchers found prostate-specific antigen (PSA) in the female fluid. In men, PSA is produced by the prostate. Women's bodies contain prostate tissue too, in structures known as the Skene's glands, located on the front wall of the vagina, that drain via ducts into the lower end of the urethra. The 2014 study suggested that these glands play a crucial part in producing female ejaculate.

Clarification comes, Professor Whipple has argued, by firstly distinguishing between female ejaculation and 'squirting'. Female ejaculation should only really refer to the production of the small amount of milky white liquid at orgasm and not the liquid containing urine and PSA. Besides this, some urologists have suggested that the presence of PSA in some women's squirted fluid and not others might be because the emissions from the Skene's glands could travel into the bladder at orgasm. It may also have something to do with the known variation in size and shape of the glands or be that some women don't produce PSA in the first place. Whatever the case, it is striking that rather than acknowledging that some women ejaculated and some urinated during sex, to whatever degree, the scientific community seemed overall determined to dismiss the phenomenon altogether. This resistance in itself reveals the threat this biological fact posed to a male-centric science of sex.

Of course, it isn't just the composition of female ejaculation that needed to be scrutinised – its function is a hot topic of debate. Most women who reported experiencing female ejaculation agreed that the experience could be pleasurable (an observation that in the area of women's health is often curiously discarded as insufficient). At the points in the history of medicine that female ejaculation was deemed to warrant serious study, this was usually to investigate disease, not pleasure. When, in 1880, Alexander Skene linked female ejaculate to the eponymous glands – two ducts on each side of the urethral opening – he was concerned with the problem of draining the glands and the ducts surrounding the female urethra when they became infected. The Skene's glands and the urethra hence became important to the medical profession as potential sites of venereal disease and infection, and not as loci of pleasure.

Over a decade later, in 2009, a study similarly suggested that the squirting might serve an antimicrobial purpose, flushing out harmful bacteria that may have entered the urethra during sex, thereby preventing urinary tract infections. So, cleaning a dirty vagina? We've heard that one before. We return to the familiar framework of 'dirty' femininity in need of scientific sanitisation. These studies, whether intentionally or not, come dangerously close to trying to explain away phenomena that might challenge ideas about 'normal', male-centric sex. Proving that female ejaculation serves a non-sexual function removes it from its equal footing with male sexual response and does away with the need to explain women's reported experience. Here we have again that palpable resistance to a sexology that investigates women's bodies outside of the male-centric frameworks we all know.

The scientific failure to investigate female ejaculation silences women within science, stifling investigations that might empower and validate them in sex and contributing to a culturally pervasive discrediting of their sense of self-knowledge and agency. If ignoring women's filmed evidence of their ejaculation wasn't enough, science and law now conspire to erase the phenomenon from cultural consciousness entirely. In the UK, where watching pornography is overall legal (with the exception of child pornography and what is termed 'extreme pornography', which includes acts like necrophilia, non-consensual sex and bestiality), its 2014 revised obscenity laws banned videos depicting female ejaculation. Given the ongoing debates about the proportion of female ejaculate that is urine, porn that shows women ejaculating was deemed to fall under 'urolagnia', a fetish for urination, which was censored that year on the grounds that it's considered shocking or disgusting. The British Board of Film Classification (BBFC) now generally refuses to pass videos that include female ejaculation that touches sexual partners, considering this to be equivalent to urination during sex.

It is difficult not to observe in these restrictions the same male-dominated standard of a sexual 'norm' witnessed in Masters and Johnson's theories in the 1960s and 1970s. While female ejaculation is censored, male ejaculation continues to not only be permitted but is indispensable to most porn. Moreover, given that videos of women being whipped, strangled, gagging on erect penises or penetrated by large objects generally pervade the internet, it is difficult to understand why basic female physiological functions that are pleasurable to women, whether we understand them scientifically or not, are deemed illicit. It is also baffling just how much the implementation of the law hinges on the constitution of the female ejaculate. Or perhaps not surprising at all, given the scientific proclivity to elevate physical, biological facts to the status of all-telling, status quo-affirming, incontestable truth.

We see here a repeat of the same heated discussion around a woman's fluids that, in science, revealed how invested researchers were in their male-dominated model of 'normal' sex. This comes at the cost of the truth of women's sexual experience. Here, too, we might ask if what the censors are really worried about is the chemical constitution of female ejaculate. Perhaps, instead, what is at stake is the safeguarding of a specific form of sexual intercourse that consolidates male subjugation of female desire.

Does it really matter if a woman is squirting pee or something else? Surely, what does is the question of whether this is a fulfilling sexual experience for those involved. In the same vein, surely what matters is that women's desire can be expressed, accepted and celebrated in culture and that accounts of that experience are heard and understood? Yet these conversations seem impossible within a culture and a normalised version of sex in which only men have the privilege of spouting, a culture in which a woman's 'sexuality' really means a woman's 'sexiness' in the eyes of an (equally unrepresentative) stereotypical man. We see here the same attitude described by Dr Gilliland, in which the embodied experience of women is obliterated in favour of a urologist's definition of a fluid that is little understood, ironically precisely as a result of this dismissal of female bodies from the research agenda.

It is also important to understand that while the BBFC might not pass videos of female ejaculation, the internet remains rife with them, not least with productions from less regulated markets. Only, as UK sex educator and nurse Samantha Evans notes, these are often highly theatrical, unrealistic performances, showing women expelling impossible volumes of fluid. Women looking to understand their physiology will find an overrepresentation of these unrealistic points of reference. The flip side of censorship, as opposed to open discussion and education, is the lack of contextualisation of the illicit material that slips (or more accurately, squirts) between the legislative cracks. These pornographic representations put inordinate pressure on female ejaculators to live up to the heightened performances they and their partners find online. This pressure to perform, Dr Gilliland reminded me, is not new. Women have long felt that they have to orgasm quickly and predictably to mirror male sexual response. When female ejaculation, like female sexuality more generally, is erased and treated as taboo, any representations that surface are easily usurped by a culture, and apparently a legal system, all too eager to frame female sexuality as subservient to male pleasure.

This leaves women feeling shame, guilt and anger. It also leaves them feeling inadequate, like they have failed. An important trend that emerges from the few survey studies that have been done on the female experience of ejaculation is the sense of the confusion and embarrassment that may prevent women from discussing it. For those who believe it to be urinary incontinence, sex may be riddled with frantic trips to the bathroom in an attempt to hide their 'abnormality' from their partners. A lack of discussion of even the little medical understanding there is leaves many women who do ejaculate feeling ashamed, and prevents those women who might find it pleasurable to do so to hold back. This suppression can be uncomfortable.

Zoë Ligon, a Michigan-based sex educator, in writing about her own journey towards squirting, describes the pain she felt before the transformative experience: 'In my B.S. (Before Squirting) days, when I held it in, what resulted was a very painful sensation in my bladder that just felt . . . wrong. Now, I love squirting partly because I'm letting my body release the fluids that build up in my bladder when I'm aroused. It's like an affirmation that I'm a living, breathing, fertile creature."[9] Dr Gilliland similarly confirmed in her study that once women had the relevant information, female ejaculation could enhance their sex lives. One participant described how, once she and her husband understood that her ejaculation was a sign of sexual arousal rather than something pathological, it became something she and her husband chased and was no longer something to hide.

We have here a vicious cycle, in which a culture of male-centric sex generates poor research based on this normalised model, reinforcing the cultural silence and stigma around the female-embodied experience of sex. This, in turn, inhibits research that relies on women who are able to experience and openly discuss sex, leading to greater stigma that harms women's sex lives, as science is unable to challenge the assumptions about the male and female bodies that exist in culture, and now even the law. The silence in medicine and culture conspires to erase women's bodies from sexology, making a phenomenon like female ejaculation almost inconceivable. And if Masters and Johnson's contributions to female sexual emancipation have not been as emancipatory as we thought, it is because they failed to listen and respond to the potential study participants who fell outside of their conception of a 'normal', implicitly male sexual response. Perhaps if they had, rather than medicalising women who did not reflect a male standard, they would have described the dysfunctions of a society that does not accommodate or take a scientific interest in female sexual satisfaction.

The male anatomist's gaze in sex and science has blinded us all to the experience of women. The scientific impulse to dominate rather than understand non-male bodies is connected to the oppression of women in sexual relationships. The history of scientists explaining ejaculation away is just another expression, captured equally neatly in cultural representations of men pounding women all over our TV screens, that female bodies are mysterious voids designed to be dominated but never understood. This science, beyond blocking entire avenues of inquiry, also denies women the right to know themselves, denies their words meaning in a medical system that refuses to hear them, instead of following voices. This makes choosing to investigate female ejaculation via the accounts of ejaculators themselves an anti-sexist act. By giving women's accounts the status of a scientific question worth investigating, we subvert a power hierarchy in which a male gaze continues to define what is knowable, and who gets to know themselves.

Sex educators like Samantha Evans who talk to women about their sexual experiences every day are optimistic that there is an emerging and more open conversation around female sexuality. Many sex educators are now very active online, sharing information and responding to misinformation – all sardonic, all in the spirit of destigmatising conversations and providing resources for curious women about their bodies. Unlike the misinformation and harmful messaging spread by certain wellness companies or GripTok-ers, here we have an example of how non-scientists can helpfully step into the vacuums medicine leaves. Many are very candid about their own experiences. Zoë Ligon (@thongria) who provides information about sex toys, produces informative videos but also writes about her own journey towards ejaculation online. Others, like Ev'Yan Whitney, emphasise women's relationships to their own bodies, posting love letters online to 'women who squirt', encouraging women to trust their own experiences of ejaculation, even as scientific studies continue to explain away the reality of the experience. Many other public-facing sexologists have also spoken out, encouraging women to squirt, and sharing tips and tricks for anyone who wants to try it. The changing culture around female ejaculation was also encouragingly captured by a 2013 Austrian international survey[10] of 320 women and their partners, almost all of whom reported female ejaculation to have a positive impact on their sex lives. These are positive developments, only researchers will have to continue to push for science to respond to and incorporate new forms of knowledge.

Women's words provide insight into the impact of ejaculation on their sex lives, but they also present an untapped resource of scientific information. Scientists will need to learn to design research that is attuned to its own gendered biases. They will need to find new ways of interpreting women's words, to innovate as they render them scientific and as important as the data produced on the sweating, pulsating and gushing of their bodies. We need to move towards a science that describes female sexual arousal and doesn't mirror male sexual response.

Just as in the 1960s, we are faced here, in the twenty-first century, with another potential watershed moment. Only now how we respond and choose to interpret women's voices will decide whether medicine benefits. This will require a close examination of the gendered ideas at the core of the questions sexology is asking. Taking female ejaculation seriously, as the pioneering sex educator Deborah Sundahl says, 'is connectable to a broadening of women's social and sexual roles'.[11] We need a sexually healthy society to ensure that not just male but *all* types of bodies, equally in all configurations of sexual relationships, are allowed to be visible in science and society. Only then will the field of sexology, and sexual emancipation, progress.

Chapter 5

Genealogies

Scientific inquiry, and so the medical possibilities available to women, have been stunted by gendered assumptions about women's bodies: a reduction of women's health to childbearing, a silent mandate that male-centric research should be prioritised, that idea that women should prize sexiness over health, and the ever-present notion that men are dominant. These roles are intrinsic to much of the research being done, fundamental even, yet they wouldn't exist without an even more foundational distinction that pervades biological thinking: the binary distinction between male and female.

The differences between male and female reproductive systems have long served as a biological argument for the oppression of women, as I have already touched on. Throughout history, the drive to distinguish between men and women meant that the findings of medical studies were foreclosed, designed to lead to results that could be ascribed neatly to sex differences. Because of this, the biological differences between men and women haven't just been taken for granted in medicine but have formed the most basic assumptions that have led to foregone conclusions in research – medical research that has offered scientific 'proof' about the naturalised roles of men and women.

Prior to the eighteenth century, the common belief was that women and men represented two different forms of one essential sex, the only difference being that in the lesser female, the genitalia resided inside rather than outside the body.[1] This view shifted in the eighteenth century to one of the two sexes as incommensurable opposites. It comes as no surprise that women came off significantly worse than men in the new two-sex model of human anatomy,[2] and from the nineteenth century, science became invested in proving the inferiority of women. Reduced first to specific organs, the uterus and then the ovaries, a woman's role became consolidated as a child-bearer in society.

Locating the 'seat of femininity' was just the beginning on a path to further oppression, however. In the late nineteenth century, the ovaries became the target of the new medical specialty that came to be known as gynaecology. Thousands of women across Europe and America were operated on to remove the ovaries for the treatment of various 'neuroses'. Gynaecology formed around this idea that certain behaviours and traits were the result of a female deficiency and that medical intervention was the cure. Not only did scientists accumulate biological evidence to limit women to childbearing in society, their biology now deemed them inherently inferior. The persistent medical interventions by doctors who knew better continued to consolidate this idea, bringing women in line with what they had decided was an acceptable norm through experiments and cures designed to maintain their status quo.

Early in the twentieth century, the 'essence' of femininity spread from organs to chemical substances known as sex hormones. The new field of sex endocrinology introduced the concept of 'female' and 'male' sex hormones as chemical messengers of gender. From 1905, when the concept of the hormone was first formulated, up until the 1920s, the prevailing – and utterly false – notion was that specific hormones were produced by the ovaries and the testicles, unique to each sex, and that these directly determined gender. This meant female hormones could only be found in women and determined their sexual characteristics, just as male hormones were unique to men and determined their masculine characteristics. Whereas before the challenge had been to search for an organ that explained the differences between men and women, now it was to understand that the substances produced by the gonads (the testes for men, the ovaries in women) accomplished this process of differentiation.

The biological substance at the heart of the science may have changed, but the aims of scientists remained unwavering. The new studies in endocrinology all involved experiments on sexual differentiation – other possible functions of hormones were not considered, betraying the implicit aim at the core of this field: to accrue yet further biological evidence for the social division between men and women.

Hormones became part of ever-expansive theories that connected sex development of the gonads to behaviour and the brain. The sex hormones in the womb were assumed to lead directly to corresponding genitals and physiological traits, even including heterosexual erotic orientation, cognitive patterns and interests. Gendered assumptions about behaviour were connected to biology to build an increasingly robust *social* division between the sexes.

In this way, hormones mapped onto and reinforced the same gendered model in medicine that made women defective and their bodies controllable through drastic interventions. Hormones were linked to female behaviour, negative traits such as weakness, mania and hysteria. In the 1930s, the long-standing practice of ovary removal was replaced with a new set of hormonal therapies designed to treat an ever-expanding list of female disorders. Premenstrual syndrome (PMS) was defined at this time – and to this day remains associated with the idea of a biologically irrational female. Hormones became drugs that were simply looking for diseases, used to treat what were deemed abnormalities only because they were female, thus continually reaffirming women's inferiority to men.

This idea still exists today with the plethora of hormonal products designed to prevent pregnancy or increase fertility. (Anyone else getting flashes of jade eggs? A waft of vaginal steam, perhaps?) These therapies show how ideas about the 'normal' female or male body are reinforced *through* biology, linking social gender roles to biological material. Hormone therapy in the male body continues to be targeted at sex drive and energy; in female bodies the focus is on reproductive activity and 'mood swings' – on the roles and behaviours that, apparently, still define a woman's deficiencies, and so, the limitations of her role in patriarchal society.

There is no doubt that hormone therapy has helped many women manage pregnancies or, for example, the symptoms of menopause, yet it is important to ask how these therapies could be replaced or improved when individual needs, rather than gendered expectations, drive their use. These hormonal therapies carried the same implicit assumption that hormones directly shaped gendered behaviour, identity and sexual orientation. As in sexology, here too scientists found only the answers they were looking for. Hormones became a tool that scientists used to reaffirm what they purported to know.

Given this history of the cultural ideas driving hormone research, it is unsurprising that endocrinology as a field took off in the 1950s, at a time when the neatly gendered view of the body was under threat. As the punk trans philosopher Paul B. Preciado has written, the 1950s saw the political rise of feminism, of homosexuality, of transvestites and transsexuals, all seeking to escape or transform the sex/gender identity assigned to them at birth, and the social roles these came with. The biological grounds of sexual difference were crumbling, the neat division between productive men and reproductive women with it. How would economies function, how would society continue to reproduce itself, with men and women refusing to perform the paid or unpaid labour ascribed to them? Hormones became a focus for social control.

That behaviours, roles, functions and characteristics – considered as typically male or female in Western culture – have been ascribed to hormones is hugely problematic. For all the reasons we've already covered, yes, but also, for the simple fact that it misrepresents the science.

Much has been written and reported, not least in the context of COVID trials,[3] on the illogical sleights of hand that have led scientists to refer to women's supposedly erratic hormones, of which they know very little, as a reason to exclude them from clinical trials. These are missed opportunities to learn more about the supposedly confounding aspects of female biology. The worry is that including their bodies will lead to inconsistencies in the data – female biology is framed as an anomaly to a male default rather than as an equally important biological system that needs to be explained. What we hear here is the implicit message that female bodies aren't worth understanding, that it is easier to dismiss them as irregular than to reshape the field to understand their bodies. Assumptions about hormones have, as long as we have known about them, limited an understanding of hormones themselves, and have shaped a medicine that prizes consolidating gender differences over serving the health of individual bodies. Binary thinking about hormones is bad for us all and, to find a way out, we will have to rethink not just the inclusion of all people but also how and when we distinguish between them.

Although the so-called sex hormones do play a role in the development of the sex characteristics during development inside the womb, there has been mounting conclusive evidence since the 1920s that, after birth, these hormones also play vital roles in a variety of other biological processes – from fat ratio to cardiac health and bone density – across genders. As researchers began to unearth the chemical structures of hormones, the first striking discovery showed that large quantities of oestrogens, supposedly the 'female' hormone, were found not only in pregnant mares but also in male stallions. This baffled researchers who believed that oestrogen and progesterone were directly linked to the female reproductive process.

In the 1930s, researchers similarly began to find the 'male' hormones in female animals. Yet endocrinologists were remarkably reluctant to reassess their binary model of sex hormones. So strong was the belief that hormones were directly linked to gender that researchers began looking for causes outside the body for the presence of 'heterosexual' hormones, such as food sources and environmental factors. From the very inception of the chemical basis of sexual difference, researchers were confronted with information that blurred their binarised version of biological sex, and equally, from its inception, they were resolute to explain this information away. And so, blinded by their assumptions, they continually looked for ways to explain away and minimise the very real scientific evidence that was staring them in the face.

This commitment to binarised hormones reflecting an equally binarised conception of biological sex continues today. Even now, science textbooks continue to use the term 'sex hormone' to imply that the so-called female sex hormone, oestrogen, is restricted to females, testosterone to males. These same textbooks discuss the sex hormones as exclusively involved in sex-related physiological roles, preserving the idea that the male and female sexes are defined by sex-specific hormones while also miseducating future generations on the role they play in human biology.[4]

From the 1950s, science, with its new techniques for reading genetic and chromosomal differences and measuring endocrinological levels, has increasingly revealed variables that could not be reduced to the binarised model of biological sex based on reproductive hormones. Slowly, these have begun to complicate the explanations it has offered of the role of the sex hormones in biology.

Intersex discussions

To assess how much medicine has advanced in its understanding since the mid-twentieth century, perhaps the best place to look is at its treatment of intersex people. Born with any of several sex characteristics including chromosome patterns, gonads or genitals that do not fit typical binary notions of male or female bodies, the very existence of these people has always posed a challenge to the neatly binarised view of biological sex based on hormones. On the cusp between male and female, does medicine acknowledge their biological existence? Have we begun to complicate our picture of biological sex?

Intersex people have posed both a challenge and an opportunity to scientists eager to reaffirm their gendered views through the science of endocrinology. The early history of studies on intersex people, then called hermaphrodites, revealed the same resistance to any evidence that complicated the biologically distinct view of the sexes as it did to the scientists working on animals in the early twentieth century.

In his early work at Johns Hopkins University, John Money, one of the key and most prolific early researchers in the field, studied patients born with ambiguous genitalia, finding that despite their 'confusing' anatomy, they developed normal gender identities as either men or women, not in-between or sex neutral. This led him to conclude initially that gender identity was determined by how a child was raised, and not by any chemical biological disposition. Much of Money's research into intersex people affirmed this view.

In his studies of intersex women with 'adrenogenital syndrome' (now called congenital adrenal hyperplasia), a genetic disorder that causes overproduction of androgens (the 'male' sex hormone) from the adrenal glands, Money noted that these women developed 'normal' gender identities despite the presence of male hormones. As the field of endocrinology grew, however, Money changed his position, feeling the need to incorporate the burgeoning evidence emerging from the field that hormones played a definitive role in defining gendered behaviours. Money developed his view on gender to accommodate this biological dimension. Now he pointed to the aspects of the sexuality of these women in which he saw differences, however subtle, from so-called 'normal' women. Among them were that these women were aroused by visual and narrative cues, while 'ordinary' women were aroused by touch. These intersex women were also more aroused than was normal (or acceptable?) for most women. Dr Money turned to assumptions about normal, gendered behaviour, imperceptible differences he needed to find in order to place his findings within the explanatory frameworks that increasingly emphasised hormones as the drivers of a biological sexual difference that was actually social.

The hunt for hormonally driven differences in gendered behaviour continued. As part of this, Dr Money and various junior colleagues conducted studies that compared hormone-exposed children and adults to unexposed groups. They found that girls and women exposed to high levels of androgen exhibited sexual traits and behaviour that were considered to be more 'masculine' than expected. These included the subjects' interest in careers versus marriage and motherhood, preferred games and playmates in childhood, manner of dress, cognitive skills, like verbal or mathematical ability and spatial relations, and occupational habits in adults. Today these assumptions might seem ludicrous, yet the more scientists conducted studies that compared these groups, the more they noted the differences they were determined to find – with the result, the more convincing the growing body of research supporting hormonally driven gender differences seemed.

What this early history of intersex endocrinology demonstrates is that we will not rectify the sexist imbalances in medicine simply by shifting resources and attention to them. Inclusion in a system based on gendered biases will only reinforce these ideas in new guises. Intersex bodies blur the boundaries of a binary sex model, and so have always presented the opportunity, witnessed in Dr Money's earlier work, to challenge the rigid binary of sex hormones, and with it, the gender roles they substantiate. Researchers today are starting to meet this challenge – which is considerable, given that gendered ideas riddle the history of research in their field, let alone their own preconceptions as people. Intersex, in a clinical context, has, since 2006, been known under the header of 'disorders of sex development' (DSD) in medicine.

DSDs are at the heart of a set of specialised fields that deal directly with the development of the gendered body. They're called disorders, but generally DSDs don't refer to bodies with functional problems, only bodies that differ from the statistical average in their gendered components. Many of these would not lead to any apparent differences in the genitals.

Genetic technology, for example, has revealed that there is variation in the relationship between the biological markers of sex, such as the genetic and hormonal, that were long assumed always to align perfectly. One such example is androgen insensitivity syndrome (AIS), in which an individual's genetic sex (genotype) differs from their observable secondary sex characteristics (phenotypes). Typically, a foetus with AIS will have a male sex-determining chromosome, XY, as opposed to the XX for females.

Due to a defect on the androgen receptor (AR) gene located on the X chromosome, a foetus with AIS will not be able to process the androgens that play a role in the development of the gonads (the 'primary' reproductive organs) and other secondary sex characteristics in males, like fat-to-muscle ratio, body hair or broader shoulders. The foetus will consequently develop differently compared to males who are not resistant to androgens. In the most extreme case of the syndrome, complete androgen insensitivity syndrome (CAIS), where a male XY genotype produces as many androgens as another genetic male would, but is totally resistant to them, the XY foetus will develop female genitalia and will appear biologically female, while they will have testes located in the abdomen, groin or labia. Until the disease was linked to the X chromosome in the 1970s, many people with CAIS would have gone undiagnosed, given that they would look, on the outside, like a woman without CAIS. Even today the prevalence of the syndrome is not known; it is estimated to occur anywhere between one in 20,000 and one in 60,000 births.

The syndrome provides an interesting model for scientists studying the effects of the sex hormones on the human body. Especially in the case of CAIS, where a body produces androgens as much as an average genetic male but is insensitive to them, and so displays none of the usual effects, researchers can compare these individuals to male and female control groups, whose genes and hormones align according to the statistical norm, to better understand the role that androgen usually plays in bodies in early development, and over the course of a life. Moreover, in treating individuals with CAIS, to maximise their long-term health, clinicians have learnt more about the role of the supposed sex hormones in both male and female bodies.

Yet the field continues to find itself stumped by the lingering fossil of binary sex, reflected in the treatment of its patients. The surgical removal of the gonads in CAIS patients is a case in point. It used to be standard practice to remove the gonads as soon as an individual was diagnosed with CAIS due to the risk of the internalised testes developing into a tumour. In the past, doctors would advise parents to have their child's gonads removed preventatively, and to raise their child as female. It is now understood however that it is rare that the internal testes will develop into a tumour before puberty, and that, in fact, the gonads are important during puberty, as they support the sexual development of CAIS women in ways that hormone replacement therapy (HRT) has not been able to replicate.[5] Leaving the gonads in place until after puberty has revealed the importance of oestrogen, for both men and women, in bone development. The hormones produced by the gonads themselves have proven to be more effective at optimising bone mineral density than administering oestrogen through HRT.[6] Studies on CAIS patients have also suggested the importance of the 'male sex hormones' in bone development for both men and women. Most bodies produce and have receptors for both of the sex hormones, although males will have more androgens and females more oestrogens. CAIS women reveal what happens in the total absence of androgen action on bone. These women had reduced bone mineral density compared to non-resistant females, suggesting that androgens are needed to maintain healthy bones. Nonetheless, this doesn't lead to straightforward prescriptions for patients.

Olaf Hiort, Professor of Paediatric Endocrinology at the University of Lübeck in Germany, has conducted a vast array of studies into the treatment of AIS. A CAIS woman, he told me, recently asked him about the risks for osteoporosis, given that their oestrogen levels are low, and reduced oestrogen levels after menopause have been connected to this decrease in bone density. Professor Hiort told me that, while he could prescribe oestrogen for these patients, the difficulty was in knowing what levels of bone density to aim for. In male and female bodies that conform to the statistical average, he would do a bone scan and then refer to the average intervals representing a healthy range for that age group and sex. These figures aren't known for people whose hormones and genetics deviate from these profiles. So, should Professor Hiort refer to the male or female average? 'We don't know what's normal or healthy for CAIS women,' he said.

There is a need for a more complex understanding of bone health, that goes beyond gendered averages and investigates the mechanisms and health of bones across the lifespans of a more diverse range of bodies. CAIS people challenge medicine to think beyond gender to respond to the needs of all bodies, to return to the foundations of the categories it has drawn and to ask whether its questions are driving science forward or holding society back.

Studying CAIS patients has also led to further understanding of other non-sex-specific roles of androgens, specifically testosterone, in female bodies. One mysterious instance is the reported effect of testosterone on the libido of CAIS women. A 2018 study was designed to compare the effectiveness of hormonal replacement therapy with either androgen or oestrogen in CAIS women after they had their gonads removed.[7] It found that while mental health–related quality of life and psychological wellbeing did not differ between the groups, and there were few physiological effects of the hormones noted in either the group treated with oestrogen or testosterone, those treated with testosterone had increased self-reported sexual desire. This is surprising, not because of the effects of testosterone on libido, which are known, but because CAIS people don't have the receptors for androgens, including testosterone. This means it should be impossible for their bodies to respond to the presence of the hormone.

What makes these studies complicated to interpret is that, since the 1970s, scientists have known that androgens can be converted to oestrogens before they interact with the body, so it is difficult to discern which of the hormones is driving the effects. Chemists have now manufactured a form of androgen that cannot be converted to oestrogen, and if these studies were replicated with this new form of androgen, the findings would be more conclusive.

When I asked Professor Hiort about the findings, he told me that testosterone can cross the blood–brain barrier much more easily than oestrogen and can be synthesised into neurosteroids, the sex hormones produced by the brain, which then work to rapidly affect behaviours like sexual desire. This has already been demonstrated in animal studies where oestrogens induced male pattern behaviour.

Findings like these again blur the clear distinctions between the sex hormones, with male and female hormones acting on all bodies, transforming from one form to another through various biological processes, and affecting a spectrum of behaviour that varies among people of the same biological sex much more widely than the binary distinction between male and female hormonal bodies suggests. These findings offer potential for better treatment for both male and female bodies. Studies such as these have also contributed to shifts in the treatment offered to CAIS patients. Whereas the goal of hormonal replacement therapy in the past was simply to 'feminise' the individual by giving them oestrogens to ensure that female secondary sex characteristics like breasts develop, now these women can be offered a mixture of oestrogens and androgens as part of their HRT, based on the understanding that both female and male bodies need both.

As we discover more about the roles of sex hormones, doctors will be able to harness their benefits for the health of the individual. HRT is not a precise science yet and there is much that still isn't known about the roles of the sex hormones. On top of that, different bodies respond differently. Patients will need to weigh up the harmful side effects against any benefits that HRT might bring. We can learn a lot from the deliberations related to HRT from transgender people who take hormones as part of their transitioning to bring their gender presentation or sex characteristics in line with their internal sense of gender identity. It has been demonstrated that transgender women (individuals born with male sex characteristics who are transitioning/have transitioned to female bodies) who take many of the 'female' hormones like oestrogen experience increased risk of deep vein thrombosis, pulmonary embolism and blood-clotting disorders, deleterious effects very similar to those experienced by cis women who take hormones in the form of oral contraceptives. Transgender women who have clotting disorders, smoke, are obese or have other risk factors for coronary or microvascular disease have to weigh up the benefits of these hormones to their gender transition against the possible side effects. Research on the roles of sex hormones across male and female bodies will be essential to alleviating the anxiety doctors often still feel around crossing the neatly gendered lines dividing the sex hormones, so that they can harness them as instruments of health rather than sexism.

It will take a push for research, leading to better treatment, to combat medicine's gendered use of hormones. It will also take individuals who are willing to take the risks of undergoing hormonal treatments. Yet this is where medical researchers like Professor Hiort have met a hurdle (perhaps of their field's own making). Another limiting factor to further studies of CAIS women is that these patients are often, understandably, reluctant to participate in studies that make them feel abnormal, pathological and often unheard.

People with AIS often feel disconnected from the medical system, with many being reluctant to share their symptoms at all. This posed a major hindrance to the clinical trial that Professor Hiort and his team started ten years ago to compare oestrogen and androgen in hormone replacement therapy following gonad removal for CAIS people. The aim of the study was a patient-focused one – to improve medical understanding to tackle the reported reduction of psychological wellbeing and sexual satisfaction following surgery. 'It was really hard to recruit people,' Professor Hiort commented. They eventually secured twenty-six participants, but only sixteen completed the trial. The intense emotional strain of being interviewed and monitored meant that many felt unable to see the process through. The completed study was significant, revealing that testosterone was as well tolerated and as safe as oestrogen as a hormone replacement therapy. It could also be given as an alternative hormone substitution in CAIS, especially for women with reduced sexual function, who as we have seen, reported improvements when given testosterone.

What is interesting about the ways in which doctors frame the problem of their patients' collaborations in their studies is that however honourable their aims to deliver better care, the source of resistance when recruiting research subjects is placed with the patient, rather than the history of medical exclusion that may have made them feel reluctant to participate in the first place. Even if scientists recognise the medical wrongdoings of the past, the question to them remains how to convince CAIS patients to participate in their studies, not how to adjust their methods and a system to inspire trust. Scientists must recognise that many CAIS patients likely have good cause to be sceptical. In fact, the findings of the most elaborate investigations by these scientists into the overall wellbeing of CAIS patients reveals just how far gendered ideas continue to drive their practice.

The project DSD-Life was initiated by an EU-funded consortium of interdisciplinary researchers to provide more encompassing care for people with CAIS and other differences or DSDs. Professor Hiort who coordinated the project told me that a particularly crucial strand of the study was its investigations into quality of life (QOL), because this is an area that has been neglected in the medical research on intersex people. QOL is a broad, multidimensional concept that attempts to capture not only the medical outcomes of care but a person's subjective sense of the positive and negative aspects of their life.[8]

The researchers of the study were surprised to find that except for social relationships, most people with DSD adapted well to their life circumstances and reported a good QOL. It wasn't their 'diagnosis' as intersex that was the problem. What limited them in their lives was their overall health status. Chronic physical and mental health problems, both related and unrelated to the diagnosis itself, presented the main issue for most participants. That this finding was surprising at all already reveals how practitioners in the field continue to assume that the pathology, the source of discontent for these people, is somehow rooted in their deviation from a statistical norm associated with gender. When CAIS patients are reluctant to participate in studies, perhaps this is the result of the persistent prejudice they sense in a medical context. Perhaps they understand that despite the new wave of attention for their quality of life, their overall wellbeing remains subsidiary to the much broader set of concerns that makes up the health and wellbeing of any other person. The findings of the DSD-Life study serve as a reminder for medical professionals to interrogate their personal biases and to rethink their clinical aims – the health of an intersex person stretches far beyond the reductive emphasis on sex characteristics.

Deviations in hormone action, genetics and sexual characteristics offer an opportunity to broaden scientific understanding of the roles that these biological components play in a body. Through studying the health of intersex people more broadly, researchers might break open their gendered silos based on narrowly delineated traits, revealing a much more complex, fluid and dynamic set of systems that, in every body, find their own unique equilibrium and function in their own specific way. Yet these bodies will not deliver their potential to shake up medicine if medical practitioners and scientists continue to be driven by the same assumptions.

To capitalise on the scientific potential of subversive bodies, scientists will have to turn the gender lens on themselves, to ask how their assumptions have limited the care they have offered or the questions they have thought to ask. In the conclusion of the DSD-Life report,[9] the authors are optimistic. They assert that the findings will have a 'major impact on the organisation of care; individuals affected need both highly specialising medical care as well as a medical home comprehensively addressing all issues of health and collaborating with subspecialists'. What they are really saying is that we need to start thinking of intersex bodies the way medical professionals have thought about male bodies all along. That this is the revolutionary insight of the first extensive international study into intersex health is sobering, yet perhaps at least sets the agenda for medicine in the decades to come.

The historical and current research on intersex bodies reveals how scientific research remains tethered to an old-fashioned, unproven and really rather outlandish assumption that a person's health is a direct product of biological sex. This is really a conflation of a gendered 'norm' relating to health. In a patriarchal society, what is normal cannot be assumed to be the same as what is healthy because this system caters to the health and wellbeing of certain individuals over others. The doctors I spoke with were all adamant about how far the field has come in treating its patients with integrity. But binary ideas about gender are insidious, the belief persisting in the medical profession that it is an 'abnormality' of biological sex, not the health and wellbeing of the person, that needs to be cured. These ideas slip in alongside seemingly progressive measures and undermine even the best-intended research. Gendered thinking will continue to limit the questions scientists ask and the care they believe it is possible to offer as long as they fail to investigate the assumptions that shape — and limit — their own practice. Thus, doctors will have to conduct some gender-bending investigations not on the bodies that blur the boundaries of their concepts but on themselves.

To move beyond the restrictive frameworks we have, scientists need to first question the assumptions that limit their explanations. The aforementioned philosopher Paul B.

Preciado made this point at a conference on 'Women in psychoanalysis' in 2019, and I think it applies equally to medicine as a whole.

> You organize a conference to discuss 'women in psychoanalysis' in 2019, as though this were still 1917, as though these exotic animals you casually and condescendingly refer to as 'women' have not yet acquired full recognition as political subjects, as though they were an appendix or a footnote, a strange, exotic creature you feel you need to reflect on from time to time in the context of a symposium or a round-table discussion. It might have been better to organize an event on the subject of 'white heterosexual middle-class men in psychoanalysis', since most psychoanalytic texts and practices concern themselves with the discursive and political power of this particular beast . . . that you have a tendency to confuse with 'universal human' . . .[10]

Medical professionals must do more than pay lip service to the exclusion of certain groups of people. If they do not, they will simply repeat the same gendered assumptions in new guises, as the latest research on intersex people shows in the DSD-Life report. Medicine will need to be practised differently so as better to cater for all people, and that shift will happen not just by opening female bodies to proper investigation, but by questioning the ways in which the male is default. And that extends beyond the bodies studied to the researchers conducting the investigations and the tools and approaches they use. Only with this serious scientific (perhaps not psychoanalytic) introspection will they begin to acknowledge the limitations of the gendered categories they hold. Only then will they begin to discover the spectrum of questions, needs and bodies between male and female.

Preciado is an apt reference on the social factors driving research on hormones, considering that as a trans man he has personal experience of transitioning, with the aid of testosterone. Medicine can learn a lot from this trans perspective on hormones by design. Testosterone, to Preciado, was not as he puts it an 'end in itself' – so not, as current biology would have it, the answer to a question – but an 'ally in the task of inventing an elsewhere'. It helped him to abandon 'the framework of sexual difference', by allowing him to cultivate an identity beyond the restrictions of the gender associations connected to the biological traits he was born with. *Using* hormones to cultivate identity allowed Preciado to push the boundaries of what his biology meant *to him*. Perhaps the same will come to apply to medicine, as it uses hormones to optimise the health and wellbeing of individuals, moving increasingly towards that elusive elsewhere. A place where hormones facilitate lives and don't limit them.

Given the slippery nature of binary ideas about gender in medical science, how do we judge – realistically – the state of medical care for intersex people then? Holly Greenberry, co-founder of Intersex UK, a campaign group founded to end stigma around intersex variations and to fight for equality and protection of intersex people, says that when it comes to healthcare for intersex people, the state of the law is the true measure of progress. She told me that clinicians are eager to emphasise advancement, and perhaps the culture in some regards has changed, but malpractice will continue as long as involuntary modifications to sex characteristics on children are permitted by law. If there isn't a hard legal line, the same gendered assumptions about how bodies should look will continue to drive treatment. As we have seen, these slip through even in the best-intended research.

The first line of treatment for CAIS patients remains to remove the testes and administer oestrogens simply because these individuals may appear phenotypically female, Greenberry argues. As we have seen, early removal of the gonads and the uncertain science of hormones can lead to deleterious consequences. Social norms, rather than the health of the individual, continue to drive these decisions. Intersex activists have been pushing for bans on surgeries on intersex children for years, but there is still no specific law in the UK outlawing non-consensual medical intersex normalising surgeries. Malta became the first country to prohibit involuntary or coerced modifications to sex characteristics in 2015.[11] Yet even in this country, often applauded for its strong stance, there are grey areas that allow the practice to continue. Some surgeries that can no longer be performed in Malta are frequently outsourced to UK NHS hospitals to circumvent these laws, in what has been referred to by a Maltese representative in a European network of healthcare providers meeting as a 'special Maltese relationship with England' and its London-based hospital, Great Ormond Street.[12]

In the UK there remains dogged resistance to legislating on this issue. Intersex genital mutilation (IGM) continues to be widespread in the UK today, with about 2,900 involuntary, non-urgent interventions annually.[13] Slowly, countries are mobilising their legal systems to recognise the medically unnecessary surgeries on intersex children as a human rights violation, with thirty-four countries in the UN signing a statement against it in 2020. In 2021, the German parliament banned unnecessary surgeries on babies born intersex, which although a positive step, does not enforce a penalty for violations. More distressingly, critics warn that parents and doctors could easily circumvent the law by avoiding an intersex diagnosis. Progress is slow, and where there are laws, these still need to be contested; but laws will be necessary in the process of moving medicine away from its paternalistic past, which given the slippery fish of binary thinking about gender that leads researchers to prize normalising gender surgery over the health of the patient, will at least place a dam, a bottom line that says that if we cannot yet provide intersex individuals with the full care they deserve, at the very least, we as a society will not stand for stripping them of their human rights from birth.

On my way to work the other day, I passed a billboard display with an ad for the dating app Hinge. The tagline read: 'The dating app designed to be deleted.' I looked at the ad, accompanied by images of a diverse range of couples of various sexual orientations, and thought: *biological sex is also designed to be deleted.*

The history of endocrinological research in intersex people reminds us how it is no small task to replace a binary view of sex with open-ended biological investigation, given that scientists have spent centuries accruing evidence for one worldview and not the other. That is, however, the task at hand.

Throughout this book I use the distinction between male and female to point to unanswered questions in medical practice. The female body is a paradigm that allows me to ask different questions that help move non-male bodies to the centre of discussion. Yet as scientists learn to suspend their assumptions about the biological sexes, to follow the voices of their patients, putting their health first, they might start to question whether biological sex is a necessary basis for treating or learning about bodies. Eventually, their questions will generate too many unknowns for the current explanatory frameworks in medicine to accommodate. As we've seen, sex hormones crossing between male and female bodies and suffusing various biological systems will beg for new distinctions, perhaps ones that connect the activation of hormones to the lifestyle choices people make and the overall health people deserve beyond the presentation of their genitalia.

Biological sex is designed not just to be deleted but also to be displaced by tools that we'll use to answer new questions. As we'll see, as we venture into possible futures for a less male-centric medicine, new age technologies – from apps to the latest in in vitro fertilisation (IVF) and from new forms of cardiac imaging to 3D-printed models of clitorises and artificial wombs – present opportunities to move beyond biological sex or binary gender, and to *use* biology to open new possibilities for the wellbeing of more people. As a tool for liberation, rather than oppression.

PART 2

Misconceived Bodies

There's no doubt that medicine excludes female and othered bodies on the basis of gendered ideas. But how have these preconceptions shaped scientific practice and medical knowledge? Beyond the exclusion of female bodies from medical research and care, how have gendered ideas informed the questions scientists ask about the human body and, in turn, the answers they are limited to hearing? How are the ways that they set about answering those questions impacted? And how does that go on to define the dimensions of biology and consequently the way we treat non-male bodies? This section is about understanding the limits of medical knowledge and exploring how we can better put its tools to use in the pursuit of greater social equality and mental and physical wellbeing.

This challenge to medical authority is not new. From the early 1970s, second wave feminists have been challenging the use of biological facts in defining men and women. Women have been oppressed by ideas about their biology for too long, ideas as we've seen about their sole purpose as baby-makers, about their emotions being at the whim of hormones, about their dirtiness, defectiveness and fragility. Second wave feminists defied the roles they'd grown up with, showing how culture and society had put them there, but that they were in no way innate or immutable. They had nothing to do with biology. The domain of these feminists was gender.

Yet in fixating so avidly on severing the myths about femaleness from their bodies, today many feminists of science have argued that second wave feminists didn't go far enough because they left biological sex to medicine. Thus medicine was left unchallenged, free to progress uninterrogated. To continue, as we have seen, with practices that preserved what its practitioners still assumed were 'natural', biological sex, but were, in many cases, gendered, cultural ideas about men and women.

Sex differences are real and can lead to differing presentation of all manner of illnesses and diseases — for example, heart disease, as we'll see in Chapter 7. Yet in recognising this, it's essential that we continue to interrogate the ideas within medicine — the assumptions about gender that we have seen shape research and practice in the first place.

Not *all* sex differences are medically accurate, and all are more complicated than the current medical knowledge attests.

The question we need to address is what happens when we take feminist ideas about gender seriously *within* medicine? We should — and must — use the concept of gender to reveal medicine's biases and to advocate for the inclusion of women and non-male bodies in studies and trials. But we need to go deeper, too, ensuring that we don't just scratch the surface but also excavate the foundations of medicine. We need to conduct a more extensive archaeology of gender. How can we apply the concept of gender *within* medicine? How can we mobilise the idea that our ideas about the gender of bodies shape those bodies in real ways? How does medicine optimise a person's physical and psychological wellbeing when it doesn't take gender for granted, returns to the drawing board, and instead takes into account the full scope of the social, cultural and environmental factors that shape a body's wellbeing?

To answer these questions, scientific researchers and medical professionals will have to turn their lenses from their patients and experiments to their own methodology. A form of introspection that may well seem unnerving, given that it is foreign to the realms of objective inquiry. Science is insecure. It knows it's in trouble. It always has been. Ever since Francis Bacon proposed a rigorous scientific method in the seventeenth century and called learned men to conduct experiments to investigate the natural world, the emphasis has been more on those experiments, on the prized concept of 'objective truth', than on the people conducting them. Science has been all about definitively knowing, and less about knowing itself.

I've always found that insecurity stems from a lack of self-knowledge; when someone is unable to confront and name their own limitations, when they deny the structural problems in their foundations, it is only a matter of time before they come crumbling down. Insecurity makes you cruel. A person who refuses to face their own failings often lashes out instead, punishing those around them out of fear that they themselves will be exposed. So science refuses to entertain the questions that expose its vulnerabilities. An open, inquisitive form of science would learn that true confidence doesn't require impregnability – but it does require that a person or an institution accepts responsibility. This means learning to identify omissions, it means making an ongoing effort to address them and it means acting upon the knowledge that this work is never finished. Once we begin to take responsibility for our place in a system, we can be free to discover that we are on the node of a web of interconnected parts – cellular, metabolic, physiological, psychological, social – that make the people of our world who they are. We will be presented with a rich, new terrain, full of possibility for new advances in human health.

Science may choose to draw on the approaches of disciplines more accustomed to accountability. In anthropology, the scientific study of humanity, for example, an important aspect of any research design is that the researcher explains how their own background and worldview might colour their interpretation of the people they are studying. This is important because the origins of anthropology lie in a colonial past where the supposedly authoritative knowledge of 'primitive' people held by colonisers was used to justify their dominion over them. Anthropologists today are cautious in the claims that they make about the cultures – whether those abroad, at home or of a scientific laboratory – that they study, clearly stating the limits of what they can know, while pointing to the ever-receding horizon of the questions that will be left to another to take forward. This is another dimension of standing on the shoulders of giants, that adage of the scientific method. Knowledge builds on knowledge and in that image is also expressed the often forgotten implication that no human can claim to know it all.

Biological explorers could learn a thing or two from anthropologists. Throughout medical history, and still today, they have continued to immortalise themselves through women's bodies with their quests for the Nobel-worthy discoveries that will make their careers – or at the very least a biological structure in their name. The author and doctor Leah Kaminsky puts it rather well:

The truth is, men are all over women's bodies — dead, white male anatomists, that is. Their names live on eponymously, immortalised like audacious explorers for conquering the geography of the female pelvis as if it were terra nullius.[1]

That is how James Douglas ended up 'tucked behind the uterus', Gabriel Fallopian went down as 'hanging around the ovaries', Caspar Bartholin the Younger 'attached to the labia' and Ernst Grafenberg apparently found the source of female pleasure. Their names live on in the depths of the female pelvis as the Pouch of Douglas, Bartholin's glands, fallopian tubes and that (it turns out the fantastical) Grafenberg, or 'G'-spot. These names don't only blatantly advertise the male-dominated and prestige-driven preoccupations of a science that has claimed to define and possess female bodies, they also epitomise that self-same methodological problem of a science that treats body parts as discoveries that are singular, irrefutable, definitive — and so does not make itself accountable for the unknown.

If science is exhaustive, no researcher will ever have to justify why he has chosen to illuminate his part of the land-scape, rather than another, that might serve someone unlike himself better. Mistakes, of course, aren't exclusive to medi-cine. Every field has its own specific litany — astrophysics stripped Pluto of its planetary status; species are repeatedly reclassified; the nucleus was considered fundamental, then neutrons and protons, then quarks. These mistakes aren't exceptions in a tale of progress, they *are* the story of progress; the real story, in which outliers are addressed, gaping voids illuminated incrementally, always imperfectly, over time. Only not every discipline has grappled methodologically with the consequences of inevitable mistakes.

Anthropologists have contended with their colonial roots by developing a method that holds its researchers accountable for the choices they make. Medicine can do the same by acknowledging that it, too, exists in this landscape, in the world, as part of society. While scientific papers are subjected to evaluation by other experts in a process called peer review, these readers are the products of the same niche culture, and so likely hold the same (often unconscious) biases. The synecdoche, 'Medicine', is misleading, because medicine isn't a singular entity, it is practised by people with prejudices (conscious or unconscious), culture, history. These individuals have to account for the ways in which their positionality determines what they know. This does not diminish their contributions. Their biases, their position in the landscape, are the limiting but also the enabling conditions of their work. Highlighting unknowns will push scientists in new, important directions. Science can know more by turning its gaze to the way that research is done. This approach might shatter the illusion of objectivity science has held but will benefit scientific research and the society of which it is unavoidably a part. In the end, we see an introspective scientific approach leads to a more encompassing science and to a more inclusive medicine that takes responsibility for its unknowns – and so for the people it could serve better. The introspection of researchers is especially crucial, we will see, when failing to do so comes at the cost of causing female bodies direct pain.

Chapter 6

Pain

In 2009, Robert Sorge was studying pain in mice at McGill University in Montreal, Canada. He wanted to know how animals develop an extreme sensitivity to touch. To test for this response, Sorge poked the paws of mice using fine hairs. The males behaved as the scientific literature predicted, yanking their paws back from even the finest of threads. But the females seemed impervious.[1] In other words, the males responded to pain but the female mice didn't seem to register the pain – or at least, if they did, they weren't registering it in the same way. Sorge, a behaviourist at the University of Alabama at Birmingham, worked with his adviser, pain researcher Jeffrey Mogil, to determine that this kind of pain hypersensitivity in males results from entirely different pathways in male and female mice which rely on distinct immune-cell types.[2]

Sorge and Mogil's experiment raised unprecedented questions in the field of pain research. And it's perhaps no surprise that the experimental design was innovative. By including both male and female mice in their experiment, the research pair was going against conventions in the field. There had been an overwhelming concern among pain scientists, since the dawn of animal testing, that female hormone cycles were too unstable and would complicate results. A number of analyses

– including both field-specific and biomedicine-wide studies – have now shown empirically that this is false.[3] A woman's monthly hormonal cycle means that there are fluctuations in the levels of particular hormones, and these may play a role in pain management. However, this variability does not outweigh male-specific sources of variability. In fact, in one study Sorge and his colleagues tested male and female mice at various points in the female hormonal cycle and showed that females tested more consistently than the males. Males changed their behaviour according to the sexual receptibility of the females they shared a cage with over the course of the females' cycles, while the females seemed relatively unaffected. There is a telling parallel here with the ways in which patriarchal scientists have emphasised the effects of women's reproductive systems on scientific studies. (Perhaps what they were really describing was the effect that women's hormones had on male researchers?) In any case, it is clear that in the case of mice, at least, if consistency is the issue, females should be the preferable default animal.

Today, inspired in part by Sorge and Mogil's work and spurred on by funding, pain researchers are opening their eyes to the spectrum of responses to pain across sexes. And this push isn't exclusive to the area of pain research either. Across biomedicine, there have been movements to consider the sex of animals as an important variable in research. Male animals dominate female animals as preclinical research subjects in neuroscience, physiology, pharmacology and endocrinology (intriguingly, the opposite is true in immunology, perhaps because 80% of autoimmune diseases occur in females, in many cases making studying females not just preferable but the only choice).[4] A milestone came in 2016, when the NIH made it a requirement for grant applicants to justify their choice of the sex of animals used in experiments. Now, specific policies mandating the integration of sex and gender into preclinical research have been instituted in Canada, the United States and much of Europe, including Austria, France, Germany, Ireland, the Netherlands, Norway, Spain, Sweden and the UK.

The inclusion of sex as a biological variable may generate additional costs for researchers and is often deemed irrelevant in the context of certain hypotheses. Yet neither of these arguments holds when we consider practically how sex would be incorporated as a standardised variable into animal studies. If, when researchers double their test animals to include males and females, they find that there is a proven sex difference, this is important information with significant implications for the translation of their findings to medicine. If, on the other hand, this is not the case, the costs associated with doubling their research sample are still not wasted because doubling the sample population only makes the results doubly conclusive. In other words, including sex as a variable is a win, win situation. It does make you wonder why scientists are so reluctant to change their protocols. It makes you wonder if there is a little anxiety, perhaps, that the conclusive results on which scientists have built their careers might prove not to hold. And that in turn makes you wonder whether it is really good science that they are defending. Whatever the reason, the striking and unexpected differences in pain research suggest that it is worth including male and female research subjects, that the total neglect of this dimension of research means that often scientists may not even have the tools to begin to imagine what they may find.

Although the shift towards the inclusion of male and female animals isn't exclusive to pain, perhaps the most striking differences have been in this area, given the brutally, hauntingly visceral consequences of misjudgement. Some 20% of people worldwide experience chronic pain, the majority women. This comes as no surprise, considering the many blind spots we have already seen that leave female-specific conditions undiagnosed and untreated. Women are simply more likely to develop prevalent chronic conditions featuring pain as a symptom. Add to this the research showing that there is both a higher sensitivity to and greater reporting of pain among women,[5] and you might begin to wonder why it is that the standard research subject in preclinical pain experiments has always been the male rodent.

Between 1996 and 2005, 79% of the preclinical research studies featuring rodent subjects published in the journal *Pain* tested male rats or male mice only, with an additional 3% of studies not stating the sex of their subjects.[6] What is even more striking is that in the studies that did include and compare both sexes, researchers sometimes found that the same experiment produced a statistically significant effect in one sex but not the other. They were able to confirm their hypotheses about the mechanisms underlying pain for males but not females.[7] The inclusion of females in animal research will make them as much subjects as tools in the research – because they expose much deeper-rooted biases in the animal trials on pain. Hypotheses in science are developed in response to previous studies. One study will test a hypothesis, revealing further questions and dimensions that require further investigation. In this way knowledge in science is cumulative. 'If I have seen further it is by standing on the shoulders of giants,' said the humble Isaac Newton,[8] expressing the sentiment that scientists work by building on what is known. This is how research progresses: it saves scientists from having to reinvent the wheel over and over again, instead rolling forward into new territory.

Only, what happens if we really *do* need to reinvent the wheel?

After all, the inverse of the scientific adage is also true: ignorance builds on ignorance. If females aren't being included in experiments, we miss out on numerous hypotheses, we never see the full breadth of conclusions or solutions and we are left with a science that is half-hearted at best.

I spoke with Sorge and he told me that the inertia around including both sexes in animal studies lies in the assumption that there are no sex differences. This creates a double bind where researchers aren't open to conducting the only studies that would challenge this assumption – experiments that include both males and females.

The solution to building a female-specific body of knowledge is to follow the observed differences in male studies, the moments in which the hypothesis tested worked in males and not in females. This will lead researchers beyond using hormones to modulate what is otherwise considered to be a common biology, and to understand female pain management on its own terms.

Back to Sorge's experiments, which provide evidence of two entirely different neural circuits of male and female mice. Pain happens in many ways, via different neural pathways. There is, for example, an immediate reaction to something hot or there is long-term, chronic pain that persists, perhaps even after the original injury has healed. Chronic pain can manifest as hypersensitivity to otherwise non-painful stimuli, as in the case of Sorge's mice. In their 2009 experiments, Sorge and Mogil were studying a model of chronic pain triggered by inflammation.

The nervous system has immune cells called microglia. These cells were thought to be the only pathway that signalled to neurons to induce pain hypersensitivity. Only when Sorge and Mogil injected a bacterial molecule into the spines of mice to activate the microglia, they found that this led to inflammation in the males and not the females. In females, the microglia remained unresponsive, accounting for their lack of reaction to the fine hair poking.

To investigate further, the pair then turned to a pain source that they thought affected both males and females. They injured the animals' sciatic nerves, which run from the lower back down each leg. This leads to a form of chronic pain that happens when the body's pain-detecting system is damaged. It caused both males and females to become hypersensitive to touch. Yet even here, there were sex differences. Once again, microglia did not seem to play a role in the pain of the female mice. Sorge showed that blocking the microglia in various ways only ever eliminated hypersensitivity in the males.

It turns out that female mice relied on a different immune component, called a T cell, for chronic pain response. When Sorge tried the same nerve injury experiment in female mice without T cells, they still became hypersensitive to the fine hairs, but this time, it was through microglia. When the researchers transferred T cells back to these female mice, they returned to using their T cells. In short, the T cell pain signalling pathway took precedence over the microglia in female mice. This led Sorge to establish two distinct neural routes to pain[9] – a ground-breaking discovery in the field of pain research which also proved that, due to the significant sex differences in pain signalling, using male mice as proxies for female mice just doesn't work.

Including female mice in this experiment to fill a superficial quota wasn't enough. The researchers *used* the presence of the female mice to note any sex differences, and subsequently tried to explain those differences. By following the diverging results noticed in the female mice, listening, as it were, to what they were telling them with their bodies, the researchers revealed that the mechanism they were trying to test was exclusive to males, and couldn't be tested in females. It is difficult to understand how this crucial difference between male and female pain mechanisms took so long to identify. It is deeply concerning and reflects just how big the schisms in science can be.

On top of the more obvious consequences to biased testing, Sorge encountered another, more subtle and unexpected consequence, which he calls the 'male-observer effect'.[10] Amazingly, this shows that the sex of the experimenter conducting animal studies influences an animal's pain response. Mice are less prone to exhibit pain in the presence of a male experimenter compared to a female experimenter, and this effect is stronger for female than male mice. Male pheromones, it turns out, trigger a pain regulation response in mice and rats. Given the overrepresentation of male researchers in science, this presents another very significant flaw in experimental design that casts into question pretty much all prior research on pain.

What all this shows is that calls to include female animals in experiments are about much more than ensuring that the hypotheses scientists are testing apply to both males and females. This is, of course, crucial in a drug market that produces medication that works on men but, historically, not always on women. But Sorge's experiments ask us to go further, to ask different questions and to build an alternative, basic understanding of mouse biology (which we might even see as a precursor to human biology in terms of changes in research practices) that in the case of pain might lead to entirely different medication or interventions that work more effectively for females. Just as in humans, incorporating a female perspective to challenge the male default has the potential to and should reshape the field, to change *how* science and medicine are being practised and not just who they include. Doing so will not only result in a fairer, more inclusive science, but *better* science.

Sorge and Mogil's findings point to a fascinating dimension of the ways in which biological systems and environments interact to affect the responses and appearances of bodies. There is a multitude of ways in which the sex of an animal, defined by its genes, hormones, oestrous cycle, age or reproductive phase and particular breed or strain, will respond differently to aspects of its environment – including the social dynamics between animals, the conditions within the cage in which it is kept,[11] its diet[12] or the temperature, sound, lighting and smells of a room.

Dynamics such as these suggest that scientists need to turn their critical minds to their own roles in research, just as doctors need to turn their critical minds to their own roles in the patient–doctor dynamic. In this case, this includes not only their own gendered biases but also the changes in condition introduced by their physical bodies themselves. No research findings will be conclusive without accounting for the various dimensions of identity that a researcher brings to the lab. This is a controversial point to make in the context of scientific inquiry because scientists are trained to render themselves invisible in research.

The aim in science is to be objective and in order to be taken seriously among the research community, scientists have to present themselves in this way. In research papers, scientists list their variables and how they control them – this is essential, they know, to ensure that an experiment can be replicated. Experiments are recipes demonstrating a phenomenon that can be replicated for and to anyone, provided they carefully follow the steps. Experiments are presented as a cumulation of physical objects and actions whereas the experimenters themselves ought to remain invisible. Yet as we have now seen, *who* that experimenter is significantly influences the replicability of an experiment, even casts into question what phenomenon the experiment demonstrates in the first place.

Just as with lab rats and mice, when it comes to treating humans with pain, scientists must learn to acknowledge, describe and account for their relationship to their patients. As with animal experiments, observation is only ever possible through the relationship of the scientist to their patient – *through* their particular manipulations and observations that are both valuable and limited.

In humans, the scientists beginning to tackle gender differences say it is not just biological sex but the complexities of gender at play. Through and through, the interactions between the gender of participants and experimenters shape the findings in pain studies. Only much research remains to be done to clarify the contradictions in the scientific literature on the gender dimension of humans and pain.

A seminal study in 1991 revealed results that may seem predictable in light of traditional gender roles: female participants gave higher pain ratings when tested by male experimenters and male participants gave lower pain ratings when tested by female experimenters. (It seems that the subjects had succumbed to their socialised gender roles even in this scientific environment: female subjects fell into the 'damsel' role, performing their pain for male experimenters, while males leant into the 'stoic' stereotype that accompanies masculinity in the presence of female testers.)[13]

Other such studies showed no such interaction,[14] while another experiment showed the same male effect but reported a higher pain tolerance in female participants tested by male experimenters.[15] This latter 2004 study also interestingly showed that the pain tolerance for both genders increased if the experimenter was a faculty member with higher status rather than a student, while another showed that this effect was more pronounced in male compared to female participants.[16] One of the very few pain studies to include transgender people showed that both men and women displayed lower acute pain sensitivity when tested by cis-male experimenters rather than female experimenters and that women tested by a transgender researcher reported higher sensitivity.[17] Another study showed that the acute pain tolerance of men increased significantly when male friends were nearby, while women, regardless of whether they were friends or strangers, had no effect.[18]

These interactions – many of them contradictory – are yet to be explained. Researchers are still struggling to explain how gendered biases, psychological and biological factors interact to produce their observed results. Nonetheless, these differences reinforce discrepancies in access and outcome of care. The one thing they *do* all have in common is that they all show us that we cannot continue to tout this concept of 'objective observation' around. A 2014 study showed how patients who doctors perceived to have more 'feminine' personality traits were more likely to receive substandard treatment for cardiovascular disease.[19] These so-called feminine traits included social markers like who does the housework, betraying the gendered view that this is a woman's role, or higher levels of anxiety, connected to the idea that women are excessively emotional. These findings emphasise the gendered, non-biological nature of the biases driving medics and scientists in their decisions – even a physiologically 'male' body accompanied by a more feminine personality will suffer the consequences of a sexist healthcare system. And they are corroborated by other such studies, for example showing that women in the emergency departments of US hospitals who report having acute pain are less likely to be given opioid painkillers, the most effective type, than men. Even after they're prescribed, women wait longer to receive them.[20] Women in emergency departments are also taken less seriously than men.[21] This is not exclusive to American hospitals, however. A 2014 Swedish study also showed that once in the A&E women were given longer waiting times to see a doctor and were classified as crucial cases less often than men.[22] This research seems scattered and often contradictory though. The challenge is to find a model for practising medicine in which biological sex is one variable among many other environmental and social factors that shape a person's pain response.

Improving healthcare for women means changing the way science is done. Including female animals and women and gender-diverse bodies in studies is a first step, but scientists will need to respond to the presence of these bodies in their studies by interrogating their longstanding approaches. This is about putting the humanity into research in more ways than one, paying greater attention to the humans doing the research and the relationships between researchers and their subjects, medics and their patients.

As with anthropological research, pain researchers also may find that as they fully investigate the dimensions of sex and gender, they find themselves increasingly blurring the categories of male and female they use to understand biological variation. They may find that they need different or at least many more categories to guide their research. Even if scientists develop drugs that are targeted to male- or female-specific pain pathways, these might still miss the nuances and differences between bodies. It might be more effective to customise drugs more closely, to take into account the spectrum of genetics, hormone levels and anatomical development in addition to chromosomal sex. This is also what the little research on pain mechanisms in people who don't fit into a binary definition of sex and gender suggests.

In a study in Italy, researchers surveyed transgender people undergoing hormone treatment. They found that eleven out of forty-seven people who transitioned from male to female reported pain issues that arose after the transition. Six out of twenty-six people transitioning from female to male reported that their pain problems lessened after taking testosterone.[23] Pain pathways, then, might be determined by hormone levels that vary among and between genders.

Pain responses also seem to change over the course of a life, around the time that hormone levels rise or fall. Studies looking only at biological sex have found that, at puberty, the rates of pain conditions rise more in girls than in boys. As women move towards menopause, however, sex differences in chronic pain rates begin to disappear. This might be explained by the effects of shifting hormonal levels during menopause, but it is not known exactly how this is caused.

Pregnancy affects pain responses, too. Research in mice has shown that, early in pregnancy, females switch from a typically female, microglia-independent mechanism of pain sensitisation to a more male-associated one that involves microglia. By late pregnancy, the animals don't seem to feel chronic pain at all.[24] The categories of biological sex do not explain these differences, only restate them. Scientists repeatedly turn to the variable of biological sex as an explanation, rather than referring to the more complex and more informative dynamics of hormones, metabolism and environment that seem to be at play.

We have here an echo of the developments in hormone research, in that pain research shows us once again that as scientists discover more about female-specific biology, they are beginning to anticipate a point at which they will have exhausted the possibilities of male and female as a guiding framework. Different pain pathways seem to be activated at different points in development and in response to different triggers, and the more intricate scientists' descriptions of pain over a lifespan become, the less relevant the broad brushstroke differences between male and female animals are. In fact, they illustrate the biases scientists and medical professionals bring to their practice. Sex and gender are tools that can help us turn our eyes to blind spots and misconceptions in scientific research but, more importantly, they turn the lens on scientists themselves.

Race and gender disparities

There is an important corollary to another under-discussed category that intersects with and amplifies gender disparities – race. When it comes to pain, just as with prenatal care, postnatal care, gynaecology and mental health support, women from ethnic and racial minorities are the most susceptible to experiencing disparities in patient care. The category of race in the context of animal studies is irrelevant – the coat colour of a mouse seems like a far-fetched variable to associate with its pain pathways, and this absurdity points to the imaginary nature of racial categories, where a set of biological traits and assumptions has been clustered together in humans to justify a violently real oppression and discrimination.

In healthcare too, myths, disparities and pervasive systemic inequities have fostered biases and distorted perceptions of the pain of people of colour with catastrophic outcomes. This exclusion is both historic and contemporary. A 2016 study details the ludicrous yet common belief among medical trainees that Black people have a higher pain tolerance than Caucasian people. This perpetuates nineteenth-century slaveowner Dr Thomas Hamilton's absurd fallacy that Black skin is 'thicker', made up of fewer nerve endings, and hence less sensitive.[25]

A meta-analysis of twenty years of data reflects alarming racial disparities in the treatment of pain in the United States[26] and other studies in the US and UK have linked pain assessment directly to racial bias, particularly for women.[27] While these inequalities exist across medicine, pain is a particular problem area, because it can present in so many different ways, leaving its management very much open to clinicians who have not been trained to interrogate their biases. A broken wrist, for example, is treated in the same way across gender and race once recognised, but the initial diagnosis depends on immensely variable self-reported pain. The picture becomes even murkier when a simple X-ray cannot be used to 'prove' a patient's claims about the pain they are feeling. We need better tools for interpreting and understanding reported and unreported pain.

A striking example of the kind of misjudgement that comes from uninterrogated racism in medicine was reported in the UK, during the COVID pandemic. As the pandemic brought to light many of the existing inadequacies in healthcare provision, obstetrics rose to the forefront in the news and in parliament. A 2021 report, published by Mothers and Babies, was widely cited.[28] Covering 2016–18, the report asserted that Black women in the UK are four times as likely to die in pregnancy and childbirth as white women. Many reasons have been cited, including the cumulative effect of underlying health conditions resulting from disparities in poverty, education or housing. Yet research has also shown that when Black and Asian women do not have pre-existing medical conditions, have English as their first language and come from middle-class backgrounds, they still have worse outcomes compared with white women from similar backgrounds.

Racism further compounds the already rampant sexist disregard for listening to or asking the right questions of women, already raised as issues in this book. And a key factor is also the general dismissal of reported pain during childbirth. In the US, studies have shown how this has resulted in women of colour consistently being dismissed based on their race and gender when asking medical providers for pain relief or management.[29]

Like gender, then, race is a category that is useful as a tool for reflection and reinvention, not as a source of scientific facts. Neither is meaningful when scientists use them to endlessly investigate the differences between socially entrenched groups – this will only tell scientists what they already think they know, reflecting their biases directly back at them. They can, however, serve as lenses through which scientists might look to reassess the findings and assumptions, and to develop tools to factor their conceptual and personal limitations into their research designs today.

The chimera

The chimera, in Greek mythology, was a fire-breathing hybrid creature, usually a lion with the head of a goat protruding from its back and a tail that might end with a snake's head. The chimera was a female monster that, just as females in medicine today, in the lands of old patriarchal biology was the fear-inducing oddity that threatened what scientists thought they knew. Mixing the neat categories of lion and goat and snake, these creatures had to remain a myth on the brink of reality – they had to be incomplete and mysterious so that the men in charge could assert their strangeness with scientific authority. They knew that taking the chimera seriously would reveal her to be more than a sum of disparate parts, but an entity in her own right, an entity that would require different methods, different scientists, perhaps, to understand her. And so, they rooted themselves safely in the land of their partial realities, in fear that if they gave even just an inch, they'd be out of a job. Yet the chimera suffered with people only ever knowing a patchy part of her, and some saw this and that it was wrong.

The bravest scientists did what they could, resorted to knowing the chimera's parts within the terms that science allowed – some studying the lion, others the goat. Sometimes they bent the rules, consulting the chimera perhaps, sometimes each other. They did what they could, edging closer, warily, incrementally, towards the brinks of their respective concepts, until one day the hazy horizon showed them something entirely new.

Today, scientists working on animals often make use of a model they call a chimera. A chimera is a single organism that is made of two distinct sets of cells with different DNA. Biologists have blended the cells from different animals for decades, often to try to learn more about how the genes of an organism interact with their environment as they divide and specialise. Taking the example of coat colour, putting the cell of one kind, say a white mouse, in with those of a black mouse can be used to test whether it is the cells' DNA coding for colour or, perhaps, the interaction with surrounding cells which determines how the gene is expressed and what colour the mouse becomes. Scientists, then, already have a model far superior to biological sex for explaining biological phenomena; not as male or female, or as normal or deviant, or as human or monstrous, but as a set of processes that come to shape the physical biology we recognise. My hope is that, eventually, scientists and society may learn to understand bodies as chimeras – as the products of ongoing interactions between bodies and environments over time. The task of scientists is to trace these processes, bodies always in-the-making, following them prospectively to see what they show us, rather than defining them from the vantage point of what we think we already know. This way, the biological chimera might replace the mythical one. The biological chimera asks scientists to direct attention and care towards the biological processes they don't understand, rather than hostility towards the mythical identities they have associated with them.

Chapter 7

Heart

When it comes to broken hearts, women suffer more than men. Society and the media may have told us that this is because women are sweeter, more sentimental, unstable, volatile and open to being led astray. Men, by contrast, are deemed economical with their love, giving their hearts to money, power, least of all to romance. But how can this be? Surely modern science knows better than to accept this? It *is* true that women's hearts break more, but not because we are unstable or volatile, and not because this is an essential biological quality located at our core of cores. It is because scientists since Victorian times have continued to incorrectly chart cardiological regions – and in doing so, have relegated emotion to the dark depths of the heart as something to be contained, rather than investigated.

The mysterious 'broken heart syndrome' occurs when intense physical but also emotional stress like grief, fear, extreme anger or surprise triggers a weakening of the heart muscle so that the left ventricle, one of the heart's chambers, balloons, affecting the organ's ability to pump blood. This physiological attack is about as painful as its emotional relative. It is known medically as takotsubo cardiomyopathy, a name that refers to a Japanese octopus trap with a balloon-like shape that resembles that of the affected ventricle. This form of heart failure is more prevalent in women than in men, especially those aged over fifty. Currently women comprise around 83% of cases, but the numbers may be even higher as many cases go undiagnosed.[1] The rate for women suffering this condition also increased more than for men during the pandemic.[2] While the exact cause of this disease is unknown, depression and anxiety disorders have been shown to be related.[3]

Unearthing the relationship between emotional stress and physiological conditions like heart disease is a tricky topic, given the sexist ideas surrounding the hysterical nature of women that, to this day, continue to lead medical professionals to misattribute female symptoms of heart attack to stress. This was tragi-comically demonstrated in 2019 when *The Times* reported how the NHS-approved artificial intelligence doctor app Babylon had a tendency to misdiagnose the symptoms of female heart attacks. When identical heart attack symptoms were entered for men and women, men were told they might be experiencing a heart attack and directed to visit A&E, while women were told it was most likely a panic attack. '*It's hysteria, not a heart attack*,' the newspaper reported, alongside a picture of the UK health secretary at the time, Matt Hancock, who had lauded the app as 'brilliant'.[4] The embarrassing outcome, supposedly based on statistical averages, revealed just how underrepresented women are in the datasets that form the basis of diagnoses in medicine – even with diseases as common as heart attacks. This is a dangerous bias that may be driving the rise in female fatalities.

Stress and heart attacks

Not only are heart attack symptoms in females tossed aside as physical manifestations of stress, it has itself also been erroneously discarded as a purely psychological, not physiological, problem. Stress *is* a key risk factor in female heart disease and observational studies have now shown that psychological factors strongly influence the course of heart disease.[5,6]

Stress, depression and anxiety disorders are more associated with elevated risk of heart attack among women than men. A woman's overall lower socioeconomic status makes her more susceptible to stress and its consequences for heart health. It is both sobering and important to understand that the way we as women lead our lives predisposes us to greater medical problems in this area, which, in turn, reinforce existing inequalities. This may also in part explain why for African American women, who suffer the consequences of lower socioeconomic circumstances more than white women, heart disease risk factors are greater, develop earlier and are more often fatal.[7] Despite overall declines in heart disease-related mortality rates over the past decades, Black women between thirty-five and fifty-four are experiencing a concerning slowing in annual declines in mortality.[8] The role of social conditions in heart disease can help us understand why.

The combination of work and marital stress has been associated with an increased risk in heart problems in females.[9] Add to this that mental stress is more related to ischemic heart disease, caused by the narrowing of the heart's blood vessels – more common in women – rather than blockage of the heart arteries – the more common cause in men – and it becomes clear why stress caused by social factors needs to be acknowledged and addressed medically and scientifically.[10] Stress-related heart symptoms are not figments of hysterical imaginations, but rather urgent cause for medicine to expand its understanding of the heart, and to incorporate this into the education and training of healthcare providers.[11]

The heart you know is male

The surreal takotsubo cardiomyopathy reminds us that there are matters of the heart that we don't yet understand. The powerful image of a valve swollen with pain poses a challenge to the shape of the heart that suffuses culture, just as it poses a challenge to the idea of medicine as objective, truth-seeking and analytical. And this is starkly necessary, because, as now may come as no surprise, the heart you thought you knew is male.

A recent UK study using cardiac magnetic resonance (CMR) scans, a type of heart scan used to diagnose and understand various heart conditions, revealed how male and female hearts differ not only in size and shape but even texture. The researchers analysed the left ventricle of the heart – the chamber responsible for pumping blood around the body. They found that in men, the heart muscle was dominated by more coarse textures whereas women's hearts had finer grained textures. They also found significant differences in the overall shape of male and female hearts, including that men had a larger surface area of heart muscle compared to women, even after accounting for body size.[12]

Even before considering the implications of findings of this nature for the understanding of complex diseases, the differences in the size and shape of women's cardiovascular systems are cause to reconsider clinical practice. It is odd, for example, given the differences in heart size and structure, as well as the smaller diameter of a woman's blood vessels, that supposedly healthy, 'normal' blood pressure ranges, which measure the force of blood against the artery walls, are the same for both men and women. For years, 120 has been considered the normal upper limit in adults for systolic blood pressure (the force of the blood against the artery walls as your heart beats). Anything above this meant the patient was at risk of cardiovascular disease, such as a heart attack, heart failure or stroke. In actual fact, women have a lower blood pressure threshold than men[13] at 110 systolic blood pressure. Meaning that when diagnosed according to the male standard, many at-risk women have not been – and in many cases still are not – provided with adequate preventative care.

The point in highlighting these biological differences is not to reinforce gendered values or even a gendered divide between men and women. It is a cue to go further, to interrogate how medicine is done, to turn to these blind spots and ask ourselves, what would it take to see? The exclusion of women from cardiological research is about more than the shape of hearts. It is about the shape of medicine. And a medicine practised according to a male standard will always be lacking.

Over the past two decades the prevalence of heart attacks has increased in middle-aged women, while declining for similarly aged men.[14] Female risk factors and symptoms are less known within medicine, and so there is less awareness among patients – and doctors – of the preventative measures, interventions and lifestyle changes that are important at the various points in their lives. The focus in medicine on understanding bodies in abstracted data and diagrams can blind its practitioners to the collective problems they reflect. We have to shift our gaze between the particular and the collective. To do that, we have to follow the broken hearts shared by groups of people whose stories have been ignored in medicine. We will have to wander.

Hearts live in bodies and bodies live in a world where the hearts of non-male bodies disproportionately carry our society's pain. Socioeconomic conditions make women more stressed,[15] and scientific and medical institutions have failed to explore why. These deficiencies in our *social systems*, not women, lead to and sustain a discrepancy in wellbeing.

It is the convenient belief that women are inherently flawed that leads us to place the blame with women rather than the structures that fail them. Medicine relies on this belief to continue to function the way it always has, to continue in its well-established research fields that elevate male scientists and male bodies even further. Women aren't inherently more stressed, nor are they emotionally volatile or physically inferior. Medicine is failing them, culture is failing them, society is failing them – and so their hearts are failing them.

The stories we are told about hearts aren't usually about the effects of work or marital stress on the heart valves. In medicine as in culture at large, heart attacks are what we most commonly see. Cardiology is an area where we find the media very transparently mirrors the gender biases in medicine. How many times have we seen CPR (cardiopulmonary resuscitation) played out in hospital dramas? A patient rolled into the ER on a stretcher, a doctor moving in courageously with his defibrillator, applying the life-saving shock that will bring the heart back to beating. '*STAND CLEAR*,' we hear. Technologically assisted genius and brute force unite to save the day. The Television Heart Attack is an extreme recapitulation of this hyper-masculine environment that sends messages about men and women, as well as medicine. These scenes first of all, reflect the overrepresentation of men in medicine. The patient in these scenes is typically male. In fact, a 2017 review that analysed how heart disease was represented in mainstream media showed that it was specifically predominantly white men in well-paid professional jobs who were shown to be at risk.[16] Which is, of course, a complete misrepresentation of the prevalence of heart disease. While long perceived as a male problem, heart disease is currently the number one cause of mortality for women in Europe and America.

These media depictions present a missed opportunity for public education, as the authors of another 2014 study on the representation of defibrillation in film pointed out.[17] All but absent from entertainment and even public information material on heart disease, perhaps it is no wonder that women are largely unaware of the risks or symptoms. In a survey conducted by the American Heart Association, only about half of the women interviewed knew that heart disease was (and is) the leading cause of death in women, and only 13% saw it as their greatest personal health risk.[18]

Other studies show that women seem to worry about getting breast cancer more, even though heart disease kills six times as many women every year. The explanation for this schism? In the survey of 1,524 women, participants reported seeing significantly more about breast cancer than heart disease in the media — as it relates to women, of course. The study also included a quantitative content analysis of articles and advertisements related to heart disease and breast cancer, showing that five times more of these related to breast cancer than heart disease.[19]

Culture shapes perception, and popular culture sends a clear but incorrect message: only men have heart attacks.

The highly advanced technology showcased in film and TV has become part of a familiar public image of medicine as state of the art. It reflects that 'sexy science' idea held by medical professionals as much as filmmakers and society at large – the idea that the best science is technologically advanced science with little regard for how exactly the technology is being used. We have seen how 'sexy science' is leveraged implicitly to justify the pursuit of research questions that build on the knowledge already held in science as it stands, to produce the cutting-edge techniques that advance careers. In the case of heart attacks, the techniques showcased in countless hospital dramas are only ever demonstrated on a male patient, totally erasing the question of how effective these same techniques would be on a different kind of body. This is a question worth asking, because the familiar cliché of hospital dramas, in which we see doctors applying shocks with defibrillators, showcases a technique that only really works on men. Women's heart problems don't present with arterial blockage in the same way, but with different symptoms and causes, thus requiring different treatment.

Changing the cultural scientific landscape

Within a cultural framework that treats the male as default, no degree of technological innovation was ever going to be of benefit to female bodies, because the stories being told about hearts didn't reference them. What was needed was a shift in the culture of science, different stories cutting across the semantic distinctions of the past. And the hero in this story, the protagonist driving this bold advancement in cardiology, is a heroine who courageously ventured into the unknown, diverging from the (electric) current of the defibrillator and her field, with the conviction that real innovation happens on the margins. Her name is Professor Angela Maas.

Professor and Practising Cardiologist for Women at Radboud University in Nijmegen, the Netherlands, Maas was one of the earliest advocates for gender-specific research into heart disease. When, in the early nineties, she began working towards a better understanding of the female heart, she struggled to find a supervisor for her doctoral research into the effects of oestrogen on the blood vessels. Many cardiologists told her that oestrogen was the gynaecologist's domain. Thirty years later, Professor Maas calls herself a 'gynaecardiologist', and has brought to light the functioning of the female heart in important ways. Much of this work has been highlighting unexplored connections between female-specific biology and heart disease.

Maas quickly realised that one hugely overlooked area in heart research has been the menopause. Menopause is a crucial and pivotal point for female heart health. Until the onset of menopause, oestrogen serves an anti-inflammatory function, protecting the female body from inflammations that lead to arteriosclerosis, a thickening of the blood vessels that causes heart disease. When women enter the menopause, their oestrogen levels decrease drastically along with their protective function, so that the risk of heart disease increases. Post-menopause, women are also more likely to develop other inflammatory diseases, such as rheumatism, thyroid problems and irritable bowel syndrome (IBS). Yet researchers like Maas have had to push hard to seriously investigate the intersections between cardiology and hormones. So blind was science to the important affinities between these systems that the symptoms of menopause were often conflated with those of heart attack.

'Almost half of women have hypertension [high blood pressure] by the age of 60. It causes many symptoms in middle age, such as chest pain, pain between the shoulder blades, hot flashes, insomnia, cardiac arrhythmia . . . These are symptoms that are often wrongly attributed to menopause,' said Maas in a 2021 press release.[20] Maas was commenting on a paper[21] of which she was the lead author, that brought to light not just the need to distinguish menopause from heart attack but also to better understand the relationship between the two. Once this relationship is understood, doctors can advise better treatment. Much of this is weighing up the relative risk factors for each.

While menopausal hormone therapy, for example, might alleviate symptoms such as night sweats and hot flushes in women over forty-five, some studies have shown that this boost using external oestrogen may actually increase the risk of cardiovascular problems in post-menopausal women over the age of sixty. Menopausal hormone therapy is therefore not advisable in women at high cardiovascular risk or after a stroke, heart attack or blood clot.[22] This is especially problematic since research is suggesting that women who suffer from so-called vasomotor symptoms like night sweats and hot flashes during menopause are also those who are at greater risk of coronary heart disease. This suggests that those women who might benefit most from hormone therapy are also those who will suffer the highest risk of resulting heart complications.[23]

These findings seem to contradict the many large studies that have demonstrated the protective function of oestrogen against heart disease. Scientists have proposed several explanations for this discrepancy, including the age of the women and the health of the cells that line the inside of the blood vessels, which when damaged, will not be receptive to oestrogen.[24] The research on the relationships between menopause and heart disease points to the ambiguity around the function of oestrogen in heart disease, and the lack of consensus on optimal treatment options for older women, which confronts us again with how medicine remains blind to stunningly vast dimensions of female biology. Considering that clinical cardiovascular disease develops seven-to-ten years later in women than it does in men and is a major cause of death in women over sixty-five, it is especially crucial that these relationships are better understood.

Encouraging research on the relationship between menopause and heart disease also points to a more general need to understand the impact on heart health of key events in female bodies over the course of a lifespan. Investigating menopause is not enough. We need to go further to intervene at key moments in a woman's life to predict her risk of future heart problems. Evidence is increasing, for example, that pregnancy can be used as a 'stress-test' for the risk of heart attack. Women who experienced high blood pressure-related disorders during pregnancy have been shown to be more likely to suffer from high blood pressure or heart attacks later in life.[25] Women with a placental syndrome, like pre-eclampsia (defined as persistent high blood pressure that develops after twenty weeks of pregnancy or directly after pregnancy), in combination with poor foetal growth or death of the foetus while still in the uterus, are at the greatest risk.[26]

Despite these now established risk factors, a woman's obstetric history is not included in the guidelines for heart attack prevention in women, nor are most female-specific risk factors, mainly because it is not always understood exactly how they impact a woman's risk of heart attack, and because there has not been sufficient research demonstrating their added predictive value to established guidelines.[27] An understanding of the ways in which female-specific events like pregnancy or menopause impact heart health could provide a predictable timeline for heightened risk in women, pointing to moments for targeted checks and medical intervention. Once again, scientists and medical professionals will have to wander, lose their bearings and find them again in an unfamiliar landscape that they must come to know. By breaching the fields of obstetrics, gynaecology, endocrinology and cardiology, medical professionals will be able to prevent many heart attack-related deaths in women, of which there are disproportionately too many.

Directing medical attention to the interactions between menopause and cardiac disease points to the general need to question the rigid boundaries of cardiology and reconceive what is included in the cardiologist's remit. Rigidity of disciplines, just like blood vessels, is a high-pressure situation, and it can lead to system collapse. Cardiology will come to a standstill if it doesn't learn to incorporate new areas of research. It is only at the boundaries between fields, where we open ourselves to the unknown, as Professor Maas put it in words that resonate with the mapping and exploring imagery of this book, 'where the pioneering happens'.

Professor Maas is practised in challenging the norms of her discipline and harnessing the multiplying power of fusing fields has always been her strategy of choice. She told me with mischievous delight how she calls herself a 'cardio-feminist'. As a medical student in the 1970s she was involved in the women's movement. Without realising, this awareness of the need to champion women's rights directed her in her early days as a practising cardiologist. She began work in 1988, and just three years later, Maas felt that she wasn't fulfilling her duty to her female patients.

'I realised I couldn't go on working for the rest of my career giving patients stupid answers,' she said. 'I found it embarrassing to talk to female patients because I never had an answer to their questions.'

By this time, the early 1990s, medical journals were starting to raise questions about sex differences in cardiology. Professor Maas partook in the discussion and drove this wave of research forward. She was met with resistance.

'People laughed at me, wrote me hate letters,' Maas recalled. 'When, in 2003, I opened the first cardiac outpatient clinic for women in the Netherlands, it was amazing to find so much resistance from the cardiology community.'

Many believed that Maas was giving the field a bad name. She has been called to the Netherlands Society of Cardiology on several occasions throughout her career, which demanded that she signed letters stating that she wouldn't talk to newspapers about the plight of women in cardiology. Maas refused, but this isolated her. No matter how much the evidence said otherwise, practitioners in the field continued to deny the existence of gender differences. Feminist concerns, doctors felt, had no place in the field.

'One doctor said to me, "I hate that word 'gender'." There was an aversion.'

Her patients kept her going – the women who reminded Maas of the importance of her work and directed her to the important questions. Maas defies the hierarchical model in which the doctor knows best and sees her female patients as partners in healthcare. As she writes in her recent book, *A Woman's Heart*,[28] in this neglected dimension of cardiology, female patients who no longer accept inappropriate treatment have been the best advocates for change in the field of women's heart health. Their involvement in research programmes across the world has spurred on the development of international guidelines.

Bringing to light the role of stress in cardiology at the intersections of psychology, cardiology, endocrinology and, indeed, sociology, Professor Maas's strategy of fusing fields is not just strategic but necessary. Cardiology alone cannot respond to the uncharted aspects of female heart health because the discipline has been shaped around the needs of only male hearts.

Another important area that scientists have failed to explore is the prevalence of heart disease in transgender women. There is very little research that can guide recommendations for cardiovascular risk prevention that is tailored to these bodies. This is especially important, again, in relation to the effects of hormones on heart health, given that transgender women have undergone gender-affirming therapy, which involves taking hormones, to enable a life in congruence with a personal gender identity. Until recently, only risk of blood clots had been evaluated in transgender women undergoing oestrogen treatment. Other aspects of cardiovascular disease have only been considered within the range of the cisgender population whose gender identity matches the sex that they were assigned at birth. Current evidence in the ageing transgender population suggests that both transgender men and transgender women are more at risk for various manifestations of heart disease compared to others.[29,30] Transgender women receiving hormonal therapy have an 80% greater risk of stroke and 335% greater risk of blood clots compared to cisgender men.[31] Hormone therapy is not so much a choice as a necessity for many transgender persons; it is essential to their wellbeing. The risks unique to these bodies need to be understood on their own terms, so that they can be advised on those components that *are* modifiable, such as lifestyle factors. This is once again a matter of following the body, allowing it to guide medical researchers to those areas that are not understood; dismantling the fortifications of the male heart to walk into the daunting unknown that, while it will change us, will far from destroy us.

Discussing transgender people in cardiology raises the important question of choice. Medicine should be about giving people choices, and expanding those choices, should travel *with* bodies, rather than myopically ignoring some of them.

What navigational tools does cardiology have? Beyond defibrillation, most of cardiology's tools were until recently only attuned to male symptoms of heart disease. It was only following the innovations of merging fields to drive doctors' attention to female-specific questions that high-tech interventions lived up to their awesome potential. Professor Maas pointed to the importance of developments in imaging in bringing female-specific heart disease to light. Developments in cardiac imaging over the past decades have made it clear just how much the patterns of coronary artery disease differ between the sexes.

That the default model of the heart and the symptoms of heart disease have been male has meant the imaging techniques used to bring these to light were also geared towards male presentation of the disease. In some cases, these only revealed male-specific symptoms.[32] Maas recalls how in the 1980s, the only technique available was coronary angiography, X-rays used to identify any blocks, enlargement or lesions in the heart's blood vessels. These images often confused doctors, because in many women with heart complaints, their hearts appeared normal. Women with angina, the chest pain that points to coronary heart disease, are twice more likely than men to have the disease but may have no signs of blockage when they are tested. Coronary angiography, it turns out, is not the most effective tool for diagnosing women with obstructive coronary artery disease, where blood flow to the arteries is impaired (the most common form of heart disease), because the reactivity of the blood vessels − their ability to constrict and dilate − is often the cause of the symptoms rather than the obstruction of blood vessels shown in the scan, which tends to be the cause in men.[33]

Findings such as these help to explain what has become a famous so-called 'gender paradox' in cardiology. This refers to the findings around the diagnosis of acute coronary syndrome (ACS), caused by blockage of the artery that leads to the heart, restricting blood flow so that part of the heart muscle is unable to function or dies. In women, ACS is more often caused by narrowing at multiple points in the artery − or a less drastic obstruction of the artery than is the common cause in men. Despite this, the mortality rates of women with the blockage-related ACS is higher.[34] This paradox is still incompletely understood but the role of the reactivity of blood vessels in triggering symptoms, rather than blockages, offers one possible explanation. Diagnostic imaging could be used to elucidate these female-specific risk factors or these techniques will continue to diagnose the disease for men and not women.

In this vein, various additional diagnostic techniques can be incorporated into clinical practice, such as additional coronary flow measurements to reveal any abnormal reactivity of the blood vessels,[35] as well as imaging techniques such as intravascular ultrasound (IVUS) that uses soundwaves to look inside the blood vessels.[36] Currently, these more advanced techniques are limited to experienced interventional centres. They will need to be incorporated into routine coronary angiography. Scientists here have a choice in where to point the lens – which stories to tell or, more accurately, which stories to follow, using the technology at our disposal.

Perhaps part of the way forward is to fight images with images. Film and TV culture at large depicts hospitals as highly technologised worlds inhabited by men, and heart attack as a distinctly male problem. Cardiology has now harnessed the power of images and is starting to build a technologised world that caters to the hearts of women, showing how women's hearts suffer differently, and require different treatment.

As has repeatedly been the case in the examples of other areas of medicine throughout this book, though, technology in and of itself will not be the answer. First and foremost, bringing women's hearts into view relies on taking gender differences in cardiology seriously; it requires the kind of innovation that comes from collaborating across fields and reshaping medicine, as well as the images it produces. It means taking seriously the psychological dimensions and the reality of the impact of women's socioeconomic status, something too often brushed aside in a discipline as sexist as society at large.

Chapter 8

Bones

In August 2018, archaeologists gathered around the excavated burial of an individual laid to rest in the Andes mountains of Peru some 9,000 years ago. Along with the bones of what appeared to be a human adult was an impressive kit of stone tools an ancient hunter would have used to take down big game, from engaging the hunt to preparing the hide.

'He must have been a really great hunter, a really important person in society,' the archaeologists said.

Only, analysis of the remains – of its bones, proteins and chemicals – revealed them to be female. What followed was a review of previously studied burials from the same hunter-gatherer societies throughout the Americas,[1] with astounding results. Between 30% and 50% of big game hunters could have been female.

'Bones are eloquent,'[2] Professor of Biology and Gender studies Anne Fausto-Sterling writes. Indeed, complete skeletons nestled in the sand appear exciting for exactly that reason, they appear to us as elegant ciphers, the bare bones of a person that somehow capture their essence. Often, though, as seen above, we find more than just bones. We find artefacts, and in these items, clues of their own. Being humanmade, not found, however, their meaning is inevitably coloured by our own cultural contexts. And that includes the assumptions about gender that we hold.

We already know how they have shaped biological definitions of sex, of how ideas about the social roles and identities of men and women have led to routine medical practices aimed at preserving a norm, rather than maximising the health and best interest of the patient.

Understanding the gendered preconceptions we hold is a question of honestly acknowledging our social environments, and asking how these have shaped our ideas about people and the world. Bones are shaped by their environments just as our understanding of those bones are and, in order to understand why bones develop the way that they do, we have to account for both. Learning to interpret our findings – in this case, bones – will mean learning to read them differently; undoing the stories, often littered with assumptions, of humans passed down through generations, and reconstructing this biological scaffolding.

Bones, like scientists, register the specific pressures of life that an individual endures. Archaeologists are best off reading bones less like static words written into rock and more like a palimpsest to understand how people lived and worked. Bones are an amalgamation of experiences and so are dense with meaning. It is the tiny clues – a slight damage to one toe, a bone spur on an ankle, a compression in a vertebra – that inform us of the life lived by the person those bones once belonged to. Remains can communicate a life spent hunched over, grinding grain, or of a life spent on foot, running and hunting.[3] Bones register the biological effects of an environment and this, of course, includes social environments shaped by the gendered division of labour that has men and women doing specific jobs. Culture shapes bodies in very real ways.

Here we can bring a feminist analysis of gender to biology to improve both the science and the societal benefits it might bring. We can think of bone formation *scientifically* as a cultural process rather than a presumed function of biological sex. Take osteoporosis. This disease, characterised by bones breaking more easily, occurs when the body loses too much bone or makes too little bone and has been understood to be more frequent in women. While in recent years, the disease has been shown to be underdiagnosed in men, who are screened less frequently and suffer more commonly from secondary osteo-porosis, which is not related to ageing but to an underlying disease or the effects of a medication,[4] it is still believed to occur four times more frequently in women.[5] This idea seems to have consumed the medical establishment and, despite research lacking into so many female-specific areas of medi-cine, in this case, there has over the years been a boom in new measures and devices showing how and to what degree female bones break more easily than men's. A success story, as it were.

Yet what we know about osteoporosis reveals all of the prob-lems of a biology that has failed to interrogate its gendered assumptions. This has meant that bone science has developed tools to reaffirm what it assumed to know about gender differ-ences in areas like bone strength, rather than explaining the more complex but also more helpful question of how certain populations develop weaker bones than others.

In the case of osteoporosis, scientists have found measures that reaffirm a cultural perception that women are overall weaker than men – their bodies, their minds, their bones, too. This perception has long existed but, similarly to the way in which Viagra was marketed through the medicalisation 'erectile dysfunction', has been exacerbated by a chain of drug company-sponsored 'public awareness' campaigns emphasising the higher prevalence of osteoporosis in women – and therefore the greater need for medication. In the US, in particular, television ads contrasting frail, pain-wracked older women with lively, attractive ones, imply the urgent need for older women to use osteoporosis medication like Fosamax that is produced by financially driven pharmaceutical companies.[6] These ads consolidate the idea that osteoporosis is a female disease. The more women are convinced by this, the more likely they are to get screened and diagnosed and consequently to be prescribed the relevant drugs.

Drug marketing involves ads but also evidence. Here we have a clear example of scientists embarking on predetermined investigations, seeking the answers they want to find. Framing osteoporosis as purely a women's issue, Fausto-Sterling writes in her comprehensive analysis, then drove scientists to develop easy, inexpensive methods of diagnosis geared towards reaffirming presumed gender disparities. Bone density became this measure.

In the past, osteoporosis could only be diagnosed by observing a bone fracture, which would lead the doctor to examine a person and either use a biopsy to look at the structural competence of the bone or assess their bone density. With the advent of machines called densitometers, however, bone mineral density (BMD) became the new measurable criteria. A woman now had osteoporosis if her BMD measured 2.5 times the standard deviation below a peak reference standard for young (white) women.[7] According to this new standard set by the World Health Organization, the prevalence of osteoporosis in white women is 18%. Through the 1990s, this new measurement became part of standard medical practice. Osteoporosis was now measurable and these measures made women with osteoporosis ever more visible.

Only what is misleading about this number is that those diagnosed won't necessarily have symptoms and might not have experienced the fractures that used to be the main indicator of the disease. Regardless, as long as your bone mineral density is low, you have osteoporosis. Also confusing is that BMD doesn't account totally for bone strength – the internal structure of the bone and bone size are also important. Women with high BMD might still suffer higher risks of fracture than those with lower BMD. The reference standard for BMD, based on studies of young white women, is also difficult to apply to men, children and members of other ethnic groups. There is also a lack of standardisation of instruments and sites at which BMD is measured.

BMD is far from a complete representative, let alone explanatory, criterion. Yet nonetheless it remains the gold standard for the drug companies as they urge women to seek treatment – the BMI of the bone world, if you will. Chemicals company Merck promoted affordable bone density testing before it even put Fosamax on the market. The company bought an equipment manufacturing company in the US and ramped up its production of bone density machines, while at the same time helping consumers find screening locations by giving a grant to the National Osteoporosis Foundation to push a toll-free number that consumers (presumably alarmed by the Merck TV ads) could call to find a bone density screener in a locale near them.[8] In this way, the availability of a simple technological measure for osteoporosis also made scientific research using bone density as a metric easier and cheaper.

The majority of research studies published from 1995 to 2005 use BMD as a proxy for osteoporosis – despite a critical scientific literature that insists that other more expensive measures, such as volume, more accurately capture bone strength and that knowledge of internal bone structure provides essential information for understanding the actual risk of fracture.[9] A medical diagnosis of osteoporosis is now just an assertion of a specific level of BMD.

The point is not that these women don't have osteoporosis or that the medication doesn't ever work, but that none of this science is geared towards understanding how or why, and so prevents potentially better treatments from being developed. It is a 'done-and-dusted' version of science that assumes it has identified the problem and fixed it in one fell swoop. The case open and shut. But then, as you may have guessed, it's far more profitable to treat symptoms of a condition than to administer preventative measures to lessen the need for those treatments (and diagnoses) in the first place. In a commercially and culturally driven system based on an assumption about gender differences, few scientists are asking what the real basis of these differences might be.

Bone mineral density tells us fairly little when it comes to gender differences in bone formation. Among other things, it doesn't even touch on the ways these fluctuate over the course of a lifespan. It doesn't help us understand, for example, why there is no difference in bone mineral density in Caucasian boys and girls under the age of sixteen, but a higher bone mineral density in males than in females thereafter.[10] The measuring of bone mineral density doesn't tell us why or how these fluctuations happen; they only reaffirm a pre-existing idea that women's bones break more easily. It is true that the risk of fracture is higher in women than men – Caucasian men have a lifetime fracture risk of around 20% compared to 50% for women – but once they reach peak bone mass, usually between the age of twenty-five and thirty, both men and women lose density at the same rate.[11] BMD does not explain these differences. There are moreover huge variations in these risk factors among women, and men have worse outcomes from fractures.

Much more important in explaining differences in patterns of bone formation between individuals is the role of physical activity throughout childhood and adolescence. Scientists using BMD read bones as static emblems that reveal all that needs to be known, reducing them to numerical readings abstracted from place and time. Objective facts that have no need of context. Only, just like the skeleton of the hunter woman, it is easy to miss the point with these readings, to let what you see reflect back at you what you know. It is time to develop a different literacy of bones.

Physical activity is just one environmental factor that is hugely significant in bone health. This is due to the role physical activity plays in the surprisingly dynamic environment of those transcendent bones we find like fossils in the ground. Before bones settle into the palimpsests that alert archaeologists centuries later to a person's existence, bone development depends on a vigorous dance between cell types intimately connected to the bones.

In the foetus, cartilage creates the scaffolding onto which bone cells climb before secreting the calcium-containing bone matrix that becomes the hard bone. The cells that secrete the bone matrix are called osteoblasts. As they grow, bones are shaped by the strains and stresses put on them by the activity of their owner. Osteoblasts deposit matrix at some sites, while another cell type, the osteoclast, can chip away at areas of too much growth. Growing bones change shape through this give and take of osteoblast and osteoclast activity in a process called bone remodelling. Long bones increase in length throughout childhood by adding on new material at their growing ends. These growth sites close as a result of hormonal changes during puberty, but bone reshaping continues over the course of a life.

What is key to understand about this very active process is that osteoblasts cannot form new bone unless the surface on which they sit is under a mechanical strain. This explains why exercise is an important component of bone health while weightlessness in space or prolonged bed rest result in the loss of bone thickness. Bones may adopt strain thresholds such that only strains above such thresholds induce new bone formation. Strain thresholds may change over the life cycle. Perhaps the decline in oestrogen associated with menopause resets the threshold to a higher strain level, thus requiring very high levels of bone stress to stimulate new bone formation. Theories such as these show how a statistic like BMD that maps onto pre-existing ideas of gender divides tells us very little about the ways in which social factors, like changing forms of exercise and hormonal changes, might work independently or together to spur on bone loss in a variety of ways across the population. The role that physical activity plays in bone formation suggests, for example, that more useful than finding measures that confirm the idea that more women suffer from osteoporosis than men would be to identify the lifestyle factors, related to but not explained by gender, that might make an individual more susceptible to osteoporosis. We need to take heed of the construct that is gender *within* medicine, and to acknowledge how this is dynamically connected to biological sex, and, quite literally, shapes bodies.

What we will find is that gender becomes a scientifically more useful concept when we use it to ask questions about how cultural ideas are enacted through the body.

Teenage girls who exercise are 'doing gender' differently compared with girls who are not physically active, and these two groups will develop different bones and bodies, as a result. Many girls who exercise will also probably have denser bones than boys who do not exercise. Understanding the process of bone formation means never assuming that bodies will neatly reflect gender – and instead unpicking how these connections are forged through biology in society.

Understanding how environmental factors like exercise shape bones, learning how and when, over the course of a life, these can be harnessed will also be more helpful in preventing and treating diseases like osteoporosis.

Imagine, in line with what Fausto-Sterling proposes based on her thorough analysis of the state of the field, that instead of measures like BMD, we look at the interaction of various 'systems' (including social systems not previously included in biology) that impact bone strength. These might include physical activity, diet, drugs, bone formation in foetal development, hormones, bone cell metabolism and biomechanical effects on bone formation. Each of these can be investigated for their impact on bones in their own right, but bone strength emerges through the interrelated actions of all of them throughout the life cycle. Key events may be clustered at certain points in the life cycle. For example, adolescent girls in the United States often diet more and exercise less than boys during earlier childhood. Diseases such as anorexia nervosa, which severely impact bone development, also often emerge during adolescence, and are more prevalent among women than men. Similarly, urban ultraorthodox Jewish adolescent young women, for example, who have lowered physical activity, less exposure to sunlight and drink less milk than their more secular counterparts, also have greatly decreased mineral density in the vertebrae of their lower backs.[12] These women will need different interventions at different points in their lives than others.

Conversely, women who work daily in the fields globally have increased bone mineral content and density compared to those who do office work. The degree of increase correlates with the amount of time spent in physical activity. It's also worth noting that though their risk of osteoporosis might be lower, their risks of other complications in the joints, for example, might require additional attention. None of these differences can be ascribed to gender or race, not in any meaningful way that explains, mechanistically, how they arise – and none of these differences is taken into account by medical professionals if they haven't first learnt to listen to their patients and acknowledged that all of these details can provide essential context within which observations can then be made. In an approach that takes on board the interacting elements of bone health in context, and their cumulative effects over time, doctors can be guided in when and how to intervene throughout a life course.

An intersectional lens

To understand why bones come to take the form they do, we have to consider bones in context. This becomes especially clear when we view bone formation through the intersectional lens of race and gender. Race, like gender, as has been discussed previously, is a socially constructed category. It has been used to foreclose meaningful investigation into why the bones of certain groups of the population might break differently.

Race is a social category; it has no biological meaning. Race is a concept that clumps together a set of characteristics that have been made meaningful through the historical actions of people. It was only the drive to oppress and colonise populations that led to assertions that these associated traits and values were somehow essential and inherent to biology. The germs of these ideas are seen for example in the work of the American surgeon and anthropologist Josiah Clark Nott, who used his scientific authority to defend the institution of enslavement. In 1875, he characterised slaves as a biologically appropriate phenotype for hard labour under trying conditions, highlighting how biology has been leveraged throughout the history of medicine in order to reinforce a category that justified a system of oppression through directed, racially oriented research.

What complicates this picture is that as these arguments then became the basis for real social exclusion, they shaped the environmental conditions to which Black and female bodies were disproportionately exposed, for example poverty or pollution, among others. This, in turn, has biological consequences that often make biological differences between these socially constructed categories *appear* to map onto racial or gendered categories but have actually emerged in response to environmental conditions to become a part of the biology of culturally constructed groups.

In the case of bones, too, ideas that resonate with Josiah Nott's claims about slaves continue to riddle the interpretations

of bone data. There is a persistent dogma in the field of ortho-
paedics that people of African descent, for example, have
stronger bones than people of other racial origins. Medical
researchers interpret their results through a racial and gender
hierarchy of bone disease in adults. In line with the gendered
conceptions we have seen, these studies place white and Asian
women at highest risk, followed by Hispanic women, then by
white and Asian men, Hispanic men, finally Black men. In
these studies, Black women have rates of bone disease roughly
equal to those of white men. This scheme of risk exposes the
flaw in the gendered idea that women as a universal group have
more fragile bones than men – the bulk of research in the field
sends the clear message that this only holds for within 'race'
comparisons. And so it begins rightly to undo the conclusions
drawn from research guided by sexist and racist assumptions,
and compounded by short-sighted metrics, by scientists who
have failed to interrogate the categories they are using.

Yet as with osteoporosis and gender, in the case of the
disparities in bone health that the medical literature seems to
have attributed to a biological category of race, once again vis-
à-vis bone mineral density, a turn to environmental explanations tells us much more. The role of vitamin D, for example,
might provide a better framework.

In one report, researchers studied vitamin D levels in
'non-Hispanic African American women' and white women
of reproductive age. They found that 42% of the African
American women in their study had low levels of vitamin D
(hypovitaminosis) compared with only 4% of sampled white
women.[13] Levels of vitamin D in both African American and
white women were higher for those who drank more milk,
lived rurally or ate cereal more than three times a week.

Also, for both, levels were highest when measured in autumn and lowest in the spring, were lower for obese women and higher for those using oral contraception. The strength of the correlation between each of these factors and vitamin D levels differed in African American women, compared with white women: *each* of these measured influences reached statistical significance for African American women; but for white women only the relationships between obesity, consumption of vitamin D supplements and winter were statistically significant.[14]

This indicates that the environmental factors like living rurally or eating cereal reflected differences in the lived experience of African American women, while different factors were relevant in the reality of white women's lives. These aren't intrinsic differences that simply exist in bodies; they're differences that reflect different environmental conditions across different groups in societies that manifest biologically, as well as socially.

The precise reasons for the differences between these groups of women are unclear, and while the authors conclude that African American women are at high risk for vitamin D hypovitaminosis, what we really have here is an indicator of how complex interactions of environmental factors, including sunlight, diet, contraception and hormones, overall health resulting from all of these factors over the course of a life, work to shape bone strength, and that we need to study the consequences of these variated environmental differences across groups of people who are positioned differently in society, and so live different lifestyles.

There *are* differences in the ways that darker and lighter skins catalyse vitamin D from sunlight that enhances bone development, for example by regulating calcium levels in the body and strengthening muscle formation. Non-human primates do not need vitamin D in their food because their skin receives enough sunlight to sustain these processes.[15] Humans no longer do.

Our need for vitamin D as a nutritional supplement most likely evolved as we migrated into northern climates where we needed clothes for warmth, where, during winter months, the sun is at too low an angle to penetrate the skin. Skin colour affects UV light absorption because melanin, the skin's pigment, absorbs ultraviolet light. It takes six times as long an exposure to generate the same amount of vitamin D in very dark coloured skin than it does in light coloured skin.[16] This is *not* a claim about biological race in the sense of a group that shares a geographic history. It is a statement only about skin colour. People of widely differing geographic races who have very dark skin colour require longer periods of sun exposure to produce vitamin D.

It is also possible that the ability to tolerate high-lactose-content milk related to an increased need for supplementary calcium as humans migrated north. Genes for lactose intolerance are widespread throughout the world, but in peoples inhabiting northern climates these occur in lower frequencies. This might have offset the calcium loss resulting from decreased vitamin D synthesis by allowing animal milk to serve as a calcium source.

It would be tempting for scientists searching for readings of bones as static relics to point to genetic differences here to claim that there is a racial difference between Black and white, but what does that really tell us scientifically? And how does this help anyone medically? Today the only people in northern climates who make enough vitamin D from sun exposure alone are lifeguards and farmers. Even those living near the equator may not produce enough on their own because they may cover their bodies to protect themselves from the sun or for religious or cultural reasons, or they may work indoors. Dark-skinned migrants to northern climes who maintain traditional diets may also suffer exceptionally from vitamin D deficiency.[17]

There is a growing consensus that the current minimum daily requirement for nutritional vitamin D is far too low and that significant numbers of people worldwide suffer health consequences because of an insufficient vitamin D intake. The importance of vitamin D raised its head again when it hit the news anew during the coronavirus pandemic as people were spending more time indoors and getting even less sunlight.[18] Low vitamin D levels, then, are a worldwide – not a racial – problem. Questions about biological racial differences in medical research often perpetuate racist ideas, while telling us fairly little, and all the while masking the known unknowns we hold.

Genes: important or not?

That there is no biological category to race has been repeat-edly recognised within science, although it is taking longer for scientific practice to reflect this shift in view (almost as long as it is taking society at large). A notable example came in 1999 with the Human Genome Project,[19] a new era of global, big-data science which emphasised that race is nonbiological, with no basis in the genetic code. There was euphoric enthusiasm for this project that promised among other things that in time scientists might be able to replace defective genes with healthy ones in a process called gene therapy, offering a veritable one-track cure to human suffering. Surely, if the revered code of life that scientists were about to unlock even proved that race was not biologically innate, scientists across fields would finally move away from their preoccupation with consolidating a social category and ask the socially more meaningful question about how bodies develop in relation to their environments.

Although scientists did manage to code the entire genome, they have since found that it did not tell them all they thought it would. For one, the relation between DNA sequence and the visible traits of a person (its phenotype) is much more complicated than originally expected. Genes, it turns out, don't really explain how humans form. They only offer a new language for describing the correlation between a gene and a trait. Scientists now know that genes are switched on and off by environmental triggers, and so are only part of a much more complicated dance of becoming.

Scientists in bone science have been eager to turn to genetics as another indisputable metric to use alongside BMD. Even in papers where scientists reference more complex explanations for bone development that include lifestyle factors such as diet and exercise, genetics is often added to the list, serving almost as some kind of scientific qualifier that undermines efforts to paint a more complex picture.[20]

Genetics are a tool that can help scientists understand how bones form, but when this tool is used to reaffirm presumed historical categories, it won't show us anything new. These explanations repeatedly show signs of cracks, their foundations won't hold under the weight of the unknown they can only paper over. Genetic explanations invariably reveal the interwovenness of the various systems at work in bone formation, as specific genes will only be activated to increase or decrease bone synthesis under particular circumstances – a dynamic that has come to light over the past decade in the subfield of 'epigenetics', the study of changes in organisms caused by modifications of gene expression rather than alteration of the genetic code itself. This too is a matter of learning to read differently.

Today epigenetics presents a framework that is helpful in guiding scientists away from the kind of thinking that distils socially constructed categories like gender or race to a single measure, in this case genes. Instead, it demands explanations that account for the ways in which environments interact with genes to shape a person. The term 'epigenetics' was coined by the embryologist and polymath C. H. Waddington in 1940. Waddington belonged to a group of so-called 'organicists'. These were socialists and scientists who were committed to conceptualising a new model for the organism as it develops from genes to traits, genotype to phenotype. This was a bold ambition, especially as genetics began to offer promises of cracking the 'code of life' in one definitive swoop. Waddington was determined that the new knowledge in genetics should be harnessed by embryologists to truly understand how an embryo develops into an organism.

To further his cause, Waddington called on the painter John Piper to develop a diagram that he believed would facilitate collaboration between embryologists and geneticists. The image they landed on was an 'epigenetic landscape'. The painting that was later revised as a diagram was not a depiction of a known reality like most scientific images, but what he called a 'visual metaphor' that expressed a hypothetical relationship between genes and their environment.

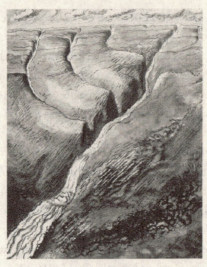

The first version of the epigenetic landscape, a visual
metaphor for early embryonic development that represents the
interactions of genes and environment, by the painter John Piper
(Waddington, *Organisers and Genes*, 1940, frontispiece).[21]

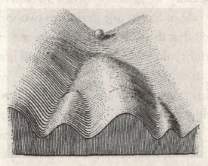

Waddington's second, best known, version of the epigenetic landscape.
The path the ball follows reflects how the egg actually develops,
the path it takes; but the grooves in the landscape reveal all the
potential paths it could have taken, under the influence of different
environmental conditions (Waddington, *Strategy of the Genes*, 1957).[22]

The ball in the diagram represents the development of the fertilised egg into an organism, which can roll down multiple possible courses in the landscape – some routes are more firmly set into the landscape by a process Waddington called 'canalisation', the ability to sustain a developmental direction despite environmental disruptions that happen through the interactions of genes and environmental forces. This is the direction the ball, the developing person, is most likely to take, but if a shocking environmental event occurs (say, for example, a burst of hormones, sunlight or famine), the ball might be pushed over a threshold down a different course.

The diagram, then, poses a question – it asks scientists to explain how the ball might come to move in a different direction by referring to the knowledge they have and using the scientific tools available. A genetic explanation alone would tell us very little – this would only describe the course that the ball has taken in retrospect, not how it came to be there. This is how Waddington framed the question for scientists in the most abstract way he could, which was the only way, he realised, scientists from a variety of fields could understand the need to look further and at the same time find common ground.

The reality is this: gene activation is a response to particular diets, specific regimens of physical activity, hormonal changes associated with puberty or aging, and a multitude of other factors. Genes cannot be listed as standalone explanations in bone synthesis, just as bone mineral density can't either. The epigenetic landscape fell out of use for a while, pushed aside among the enthusiasm for the Human Genome Project. Now it is coming back, asking scientists to read genes as part of a landscape. The nature of a metaphor is that it will never capture the truth in any definitive sense, remains open-ended and, for that reason, its meaning is inexhaustible. Scientists are challenged to continue to find new approaches to understanding the same broad hypothetical relationship, and they can be as creative in how they do this and who they choose to work with as the painting that inspired them to do so. The landscape works for bone formation, too, as a space for scientists from various fields to congregate and find their way together, as they develop new readings of the poetry of bones that echoes across the canalised canyons, through time.

Bones are eloquent reminders of the ways in which our bodies are embedded in our environment. We find them, years after a biological life has ended, nestled in the dust, a unique script revealing the life of their owner; discernible from yet dependent on the ground that holds them. The same is true for 'living' bones. Just think how much more knowledge can be found if we learn to read bones in living bodies with the same mindset an archaeologist uses to approach a site, learn how to assess the impact of lifestyle on an individual basis and how to interpret the way this interacts with their biology. Thus, a more complex understanding of bone formation is not just good science, it is also a vital exercise in humanity.

Chapter 9

Cancer

Building a gender-inclusive medicine is not just a question of better representation. While it is important that researchers and medical professionals who are women are adequately represented in their fields, or that female bodies are included in clinical trials, as we've seen, gender bias is pervasive in the very ideas that have shaped medical fields, from the questions scientists ask to the assumptions they make. These are the real consequences of gender bias in medicine – and they are sticky and insidious.

One of these assumptions, most obviously exemplified in the image of a man penetrating a woman, as we saw in Chapter 4 on sexology, built into the way medicine is done, is a power discrepancy between doctor and patient that despite steps in the right direction in modern medicine still positions the patient as deferent and the doctor as the ultimate decision maker. As we'll see in this chapter, this power relationship extends to scientific research in society at large. Here, too, a few experts make decisions about research agendas that affect women, that even make use of their body material without involving them in these decisions. This is a logical extension of the paternalistic model of medical decision making. In this chapter, we follow a troubling strand of the history of cancer research to question who benefits from scientific research, who sacrifices, whose contributions are valued – and so, ultimately, who gets a say.

In 2017, the artist Kadir Nelson, commissioned by HBO, immortalised a certain Henrietta Lacks in a portrait that he titled *The Mother of Modern Medicine*. The portrait hangs in pride of place, alongside America's other greats, in the Smithsonian National Portrait Gallery in Washington DC, including those of the scientists who have contributed to a proud history of the US at the forefront of medical advancement. Only Lacks wasn't a scientist, but a patient. A patient who, at the dawn of a new science of stem cells, also became a very generous benefactor, contributing to major medical innovations. Without her knowledge or consent.

Henrietta Lacks had already been immortalised long before her portrait was commissioned. Not in the stately setting at the heart of the country's capital, but, instead, in laboratories across the world where scientists used the cells her doctor at Johns Hopkins Hospital had taken from her in the 1950s, while treating her for cervical cancer. These doctors donated a sample of this tissue to research without Lacks' – or after her death, her family's – knowledge or consent. An African American woman, Lacks died, aged twenty-one, in 1951, and her cells turned out to have an extraordinary capacity to survive and replicate compared to the ordinary cells that you or I might have which would eventually cease to have the ability to replicate past a certain point.

On discovering this immortality, researchers shared Lacks' cells with labs across the world – and they proved incredibly useful. Research previously limited by the availability of tissue samples now had at its disposal an infinitely dividing set of cells, an immortal cell line, that researchers could test their hypotheses on. The so-called HeLa cells became the work-horse of biological research. Lacks' cells have been used in research that has led to in vitro fertilisation, as well as being central to cancer, immunology and infectious disease research. Most recently, Henrietta Lacks' cell line was used in the research for vaccines against COVID.[1]

In Nelson's painting, Lacks stands serenely smiling, wearing a deep red dress, a bright yellow hat hovering halo-like around her head. Her hands are clasped around a Bible that she holds across the place of her womb – that seat of motherhood in more ways than one, as this was also the site of her cancer and so the birthplace of the immortal cell line. The wallpaper behind her, which stretches across the frame, is a repeated hexagonal pattern, a design containing the 'flower of life', an ancient symbol of immortality and exponential growth – both of which characterise her mysterious immortal cells. This is a picture of the saintliness of motherhood in the age of high-tech science.

The strategic function of the portrait, however, the gallery's painting and sculpture curator Dorothy Moss tells us, is to invoke the darker side of medical advancement, to spark a conversation about 'the people who have made a significant impact on science yet have been left out of history'.[2] If you take the time to look at the painting of a gleaming paragon of virtue which hangs in a gallery amid pioneers and visionaries, the signs of that forgotten history are subtle at best. You have to look hard, beyond the familiar virtue-washing of a woman and her maternal nature, for the cost of her birthing that cell line (and the infinite possibilities for reproduction that it spawned) to Henrietta's own life. Two of her dress buttons are missing, a reference, the painter writes, to 'the cells taken from her body without her knowledge'. The pearls around her neck are veiled, ladylike ciphers of the 'aggressive cancer that took her life'. These gaps are the breadcrumbs coaxing us down a path that will tell the story of how Henrietta's marginalisation in society was exploited in the name of science. The signs are there, but they fade amid the overpowering force of the story of high-tech scientific advancement we know. (Perhaps this is an apt reminder of the difficulty of piecing together that history in a world alight with uncritical reverence for science?)

Perhaps the image is slightly frayed around the edges, but ultimately, when we look into the kind eyes of this picture-perfect woman, we see a martyr whose sacrifice was well worthwhile considering the glittering advances it facilitated. We might even be forgiven for misreading here in this reassuring retelling a story of a woman who had a choice, who willingly gave consent. This, however, was not the case.

Henrietta Lacks' low status was exploited in a US research and healthcare system that ranks white male bodies in labs above white female ones, and white female over Black male, and Black male over Black female. This intersectional oppression put Henrietta at the mercy of the medical men in power in terms of clinical decisions about the treatment of her cancer at the time, as well as how her cells were ultimately used. The options available to Lacks at every stage in this spiralling trajectory were limited. The hospital where she was treated and her cells collected was one of the only medical facilities that treated Black people in the area.

When researchers and then biotechnology companies and then other companies profited from Lacks' cells, none of this money went back to Lacks or her family. For decades after her death, scientists and doctors repeatedly failed to ask for consent when they revealed Lacks' name publicly, shared her medical records with the media or even published her cells' genome online.[3] The total disregard for Lacks' own sense of agency started in the doctor's consultation room while she was alive, but repeated itself in the decisions made about her body parts once they left the clinic and entered the laboratory, and the world. Science operated in such a way that it could extract the material it needed from Henrietta Lacks' body, while failing to help her in her body. Science continues to allow certain kinds of bodies to be exploited in the service of a scientific advancement that doesn't necessarily benefit them, and its implications extend far beyond the case of Lacks and her family.

Patients in any clinic are to an extent also human guinea pigs. Medicine is never fool-proof, and bodies vary. When doctors prescribe medicine that has gone through extensive clinical trials, there is a possibility that it might not work, have harmful side effects or at worst exacerbate the problem. Yet given the biases in medicine that we have seen, this is far truer for some than for others – some patients are cast as research subjects, others as patients. Some people get the treatment they need more often than others, while these others find themselves contributing inordinately, often involuntarily, as research subjects through an unsystematic trial-and-error of treatments that aren't designed for them. Lacks' case shows us how, in the era of modern medicine, where many treatments rely on the same bodily material as research does, these schisms are recapitulated in unfamiliar, increasingly fractured trajectories that span the globe.

Body tissues flow between continents, as we'll see, predominantly from economically disadvantaged areas to advantaged ones. Just as in the traditional scheme of medicine, women are unprotected but essential contributors to an increasingly globalised medical system that continues to benefit the same white and male elite. The case of Lacks reminds us once again that the powers of high-tech science do not flow evenly, that social interventions are often much more important in ensuring that medicine serves the needs of the subjects it relies on to fuel its now global machine.

The relationship between scientists and the Lacks family has evolved in recent times. In 2013, two representatives from the NIH worked with some of Lacks' descendants to negotiate controlled access for biomedical researchers to the whole genome data of HeLa cells, in what the NIH called a 'landmark agreement' that 'exemplifies NIH's continued commitment to seeing research participants as partners in the research enterprise'.[4] The family has been supportive overall of continued biomedical research using the cells, given the medical benefits they can bring to wide populations, and so it is not surprising to me that this agreement was reached.

In the report on the collaborative process though, the authors claim to have addressed the family's concerns about issues like consent and privacy in their discussions.[5] Only, on reading about their methodology, I find that the family were, in fact, only presented with three options for the full HeLa sequence data: first, to make the entire sequence freely available; second, to offer controlled access through a data base; third, to withhold the sequence from researchers altogether.

I am sceptical about this rendition of a so-called partnership in research enterprise, in which a family who, decades after their ancestor's cells were taken, used, the results even published without their consent, were presented with three options.

These determined by the very scientists who seemed to hold all the knowledge of the scientific possibilities available and who had the power to withhold all the possibilities they deemed irrelevant. Based on these choices, the family selected the happy middle ground.

I don't think this is the kind of broad, imaginative or inclusive discussion that we need in order to rethink who benefits from biomedical research and how. I feel the family would have needed much more information to make an informed decision; to come up with new options in discussion with the scientists. Giving underrepresented populations a voice in science will take a more radical overhaul than a neat and tidy 'landmark agreement' designed to paper over yet more cracks.

That said, I am pleased that the discussions took place, yet I remain sceptical about the real change in power balances between the patient/research subject and doctor/scientist they represent. Not least because I know that beyond the token case Lacks has come to represent for certain medical institutions, women continue to contribute disproportionately to the medical research with their biological material – and the demands of this medical system build on and exacerbate other forms of exploitation.

No one could have anticipated the medical advances that flowed from the discovery of stem cells: from treatments for polio, blood cancer and sickle cell anaemia, to cancer diagnosis methods and a better understanding of ageing. Indeed, some of these advances benefit women specifically today: the HeLa line was famously used to develop the HPV vaccine to treat cervical cancer.

Yet while some of these developments may have advanced the health of some women, they have also come at the cost of women still marginalised in a global medical industry that relies on the uncompensated, often unrecognised contributions of women's body cells, tissues and parts.

The invisible woman

Women are essential contributors to the modern booming stem cell and regenerative medicine industries. These are new fields of biomedical research that are rapidly expanding throughout the developed and some developing economies – the UK, North America, Western Europe, India and China. Women, in these fields, are the primary tissue donors, because sourcing and cultivating stem cells requires high volumes of human embryos, eggs, foetal tissue and umbilical cord blood. Yet while the system relies on their body parts, women them-selves, as in other areas of medicine, often remain invisible. Extracting research material is taxing on the female body, it involves physically demanding protocols, usually in a medical context, like super-ovulation (a technique used in assisted reproduction using fertility medications to induce multiple ovulations, rather than the standard one a month, at once), IVF, pregnancy termination or birthing. Yet neither the process of donation nor the products themselves are typically valued as the products of intensive labour.

Much of the time, this material is framed as 'surplus' or 'waste' by medical professionals and scientists. Embryos extracted and not used in IVF are, for example, called 'spare', implying that they'd go to waste if not donated to research. 'Poor-quality' eggs not suitable for IVF are 'waste' products and the decision about whether to donate these to research is often framed as a moral obligation, rather than as a choice

– women made to feel selfish to deny others the generative powers of the material that is no longer of use to them. The silent suffering of women is thus normalised; their physical labour expected.

It isn't difficult to see how biomedical harvesting builds on the age-old expectations of the childbearing woman. The hours, and biological and psychological contortions required to make these so-called donations are on a par with those required to hold down any desk job, and they arguably add far more value to the global economy (be that as a new generation of labourers or as immortal biological material with infinite potential for research and medical treatment), yet somehow in none of these framings is the woman's biological, psychological or temporal investment valued, let alone compensated; her contributions are taken for granted, as they always were.

Not only are their biological contributions expected, but women don't have a say in how their biological material is used. Women's silence, as we have seen in the areas of gynaecology, obstetrics or prolapse, often stems from shame. This shame is implicit, and not always obvious to medical professionals, but biomedicine does capitalise, however inadvertently, on women's sense of moral shortcoming to coerce them into donating material for free. In the UK, for example, foetal material has been harvested from abortions since they were decriminalised in 1967. Women planning abortions are asked for consent prior to their procedures, but the current guidelines governing practice mean that women receive next to no information about the kind of research involved. Thus there is an implicit judgement: that donating foetal tissue to stem cell research is a form of redemption, making valuable use of something that would otherwise be only shameful waste. A woman, having failed as a baby-maker, can at least go some way to fulfilling her duty by contributing to the future health of society.

Cord blood donations are procured according to a similar logic, in which companies under names like Pluristem or Cordlife use advertising to solicit pregnant women to open private cord blood accounts for their children. Here, the responsibility of the woman as a baby-maker is again leveraged to imply that it is moral to contribute bodily material, and irresponsible not to do so. The blood is collected during birth and the account is then retained for an annual fee. The blood is available in case a child or compatible family member requires treatment for a blood disorder or for conditions that may become treatable as stem cell therapies develop. Mothers invest in the future of their children by investing in the future of regenerative medicine through the equivalent of a biological form of investment in a commercial bank, which goes on to generate profit from their financial and biological investments in the forms of new monetised tools and cures.[6]

When their decisions are presented as moral imperatives or as redemptive acts, can we really consider women to be willing participants in biomedical research? Are their contributions really donations or stolen goods? This question becomes even more pressing when we look at the global inequalities of women's contributions of biological material to biomedicine. There are instances, for example, where impoverished women in developing nations are recruited into risky procedures for minimal fees. While the economic value of a woman's contribution to research is financially acknowledged, in general, she is inadequately compensated in a medical system that takes advantage of existing socioeconomic inequalities to procure the valuable biological material needed to sustain its non-stop, ever-proliferating research.

Women can, for example, supplement their income through superovulation to donate eggs or negotiate a free course of IVF in exchange for the 'spare' embryos that will be given to stem cell research. A global market has made selling eggs a viable source of income for some women already engaged in other forms of female service labour like domestic work or sex work. Women in Eastern Europe may, for example, sell their eggs to infertile couples in more heavily regulated systems – such as the UK, where it is not possible to produce or source them at home – as well as for use in stem cell research. There are companies that broker these deals.

In the US, where eggs can be sold on an entirely unregulated market, African American and Hispanic women often sell to research, where they will have more success than the reproductive market which favours fair-skinned women. Women from lower socioeconomic backgrounds who perhaps have had more limited access to education will similarly find this a viable option when fertility clinics favour the eggs of women with high-level degrees.[7]

This modern global stem cell and regenerative medicine industry exacerbates existing inequalities where certain bodies perform underpaid or unpaid labour while others reap the benefits of modern, advanced medicine. There are many women in comparable positions to Henrietta Lacks today, whose contributions to medicine should not be glorified but problematised, because they aren't made in open acknowledgement of the value of their contributions, nor with any critical interrogation of the value of that research to them.

Not only do researchers hold the power to decide how material is used, to restrict the 'choice' of potential uses before a participant is ever consulted, they also operate within a system that is inherently coercive, that casts a moral judgement, that demands that we all contribute to scientific progress – a moral cause that is in itself never interrogated. Only the gender disparities we have already seen in this book show that scientific progress doesn't always benefit those whose bodies work hardest for it. Should individuals really feel obligated to contribute to the progress of a science that does not serve them?

It's not all bad news though.

In many ways, stem cell research has led to improved understanding and treatments for women. The cervical cancer that spawned HeLa cells in the 1950s was used in 1984 to show how the presence of HPV can lead to certain types of cervical cancer. The researchers cloned the HeLa cells, allowing them to detect the presence of the virus in the DNA.[8] The discovery of HPV led to the development of one of the first anti-cancer vaccines, which, as we have seen, has been tremendously influential given that most types of cervical cancer are caused by HPV. It has led to an 80% reduction in HPV among sixteen- to twenty-one-year-old women worldwide. The discovery tackled the cancer that killed Henrietta Lacks and birthed the HeLa stem cell line in the first place and, in doing so, went some way to ensuring that the flow of scientific research was directed back into those areas that mattered to the bodies who enabled it.

Would it be fair to say that the story has finally come full circle?

Not entirely.

For one, the implementation of the HPV vaccine maps onto global inequalities, once again limiting the benefits it can bring to already socioeconomically disadvantaged populations. As of 2020, less than a quarter of low-income countries had introduced the HPV vaccine into their national immunisation schedules, while more than 85% of high-income countries had done so. There are similar disparities for cervical cancer screening programmes.[9] The question of how the HPV vaccine has been distributed and integrated into healthcare reveals that it is a milestone for only some women's health.

For HeLa cells to deliver on their full potential they can't only be used as a band-aid that permits business to continue in much the same way. They need to be used as a tool for a more radical organisational and social overhaul like I have described in this book – to redraw the map of the medical landscape. Stem cells flowed from Henrietta Lacks' womb, connecting the birth of a scientifically 'sexy', high-tech research field directly to this woman's gynaecology. This conceptual link should encourage scientists to re-evaluate the traditional boundaries between fields, to see that gynaecology is a scientifically exciting area and to understand that it pertains to all the other male-dominated fields of science they thought they knew.

That's not to say there isn't reason to be hopeful; we'll see examples of the research finally redrawing these disciplinary boundaries in the final, future-facing section of this book. In the case of the history of the HPV vaccine, however, we have a bleaker story. The HPV vaccine may be good for cervical cancer, but its uncritical implementation has meant that, once again, this promising medical intervention has been mapped onto old sexist ideas, meaning that scientists and medical professionals have missed an opportunity to right the historical wrongs that stripped women like Henrietta Lacks of their agency, in any real way.

The history of HPV treatment is an interesting example of the ways in which sexism is bad for medicine. Although typically characterised as a woman's disease, HPV is sexually transmitted, meaning that both men and women can contract it.[10] Figures show that 85% of women and 91% of men with at least one sexual partner from the opposite sex will contract HPV infection during their lifetime.[11] In studies on heterosexual transmission, males are actually *more* likely to have HPV in their lifetime and be the recipients of HPV than women.[12] Yet somehow HPV has come to be framed as a 'female disease'.

The 'feminisation' of HPV builds on the belief, also reflected in the attitudes we have seen towards their bodily donations, that women are solely responsible for reproduction and, by extension, for reproductive healthcare in heterosexual partnerships. In the public health campaigns and marketing around HPV, reproduction is once again solely a woman's domain.[13] Women are expected to go for screening (HPV screening is not widely available for men) for a disease that men are in fact slightly more likely to contract. The responsibility, but also that sticky and familiar stigma and shame, is directed to women, not men, as both the hosts *and* transmitters of HPV.[14] These gendered divisions of blame and responsibility harm everyone.

Women, burdened with screening and treatment of HPV-related diseases, are once again assigned a specific role that defines the limitations of their medical needs and are shamed into submission for good measure. This status quo, as we have seen, also does little to challenge scientists to explore new avenues of inquiry in order to address the needs of these silenced patients. At the same time, men are not receiving the

HPV prevention they need – or understand the risk of cancer that results from infection.

Gender bias harms us all

Gender bias in medicine doesn't just harm women. If it is bad science and bad medicine, it harms us all. The gendered role division when it comes to cervical cancer extends to a more general sense of responsibility reflected in women's attitudes towards preventative healthcare. In this case, again, this harms the health of men. It is, for example, evidenced in their attitudes towards screening for most forms of cancer. Men have higher cancer mortality rates across the board compared to women.[15]

The 2013 study[16] of attitudes towards screening among adults in New York, Maryland and Puerto Rico showed that while only 5% of women had never attended a cancer screening in their lives, by comparison, this was an astonishing 41% for men. Men were also less willing to participate in cancer screening and in skin cancer exams. It was not clear whether this was out of lack of perceived need or some form of anticipated discomfort around the procedure. Once doctors explained what was involved, however, men were more willing to attend. Apparently, men lack the information needed to make decisions about screening, and so to take their share of responsibility for our population's health. Medical professionals do not consistently provide this information, and this reflects the societal attitude that somehow, preventative healthcare behaviours are not something that needs to be expected from men.

The patriarchal model of medicine in which experts hold ultimate decision-making power disarms male patients too. All patients and non-experts will suffer as long as information is funnelled to them through a gendered lens. The case of Henrietta Lacks, of women who 'donate' bodily material, and the men who do not have the information they need to make decisions about screening, are all part of that same patriarchal system. Once again, the information shared with patients is shaped by a set of assumptions about gender roles – of scientist and patient, of man and woman – and this omits the information that would give them choice.

We need to think about the implementation of scientific advances as much as their direct medical benefits. On the surface, the HPV vaccine seems to do some work to redress the inequity that led Henrietta Lacks to birth a new scientific field while herself receiving subpar support. Yet the broader social conditions into which the vaccine was introduced reinforce women's subjugation in the medical system and so, after all, could end up harming their health.

In order for stem cells to fulfil their healthcare potential, to help all bodies, we need to use them much more creatively in order to shift the way decisions are made in research. As with HPV, the stem cell industry makes reproduction everybody's – not just women's – business. Stem cells flow from fertility treatment and reproductive care to be used to heal bodies, create body parts and sex cells, fuelling a global, interconnected scientific industry involving patients, scientists, businesses and medical practitioners. This research makes direct use, disproportionate use, of female body tissues and women need a say in how their own body material is used. These flows blur the boundaries between labs and clinics, research and care, raising questions we should have been asking all along about the role of patients in decision making about scientific research. Asking a patient for consent to use their cells for research isn't enough. Paying them for their contributions isn't enough.[17] Now that the lab and clinic are increasingly connected, the goals of medicine need to go beyond optimising individual preferences for treatment (although this would be a good start). We also need to consider how the biological materials extracted in clinics can be used to generate socially valuable scientific knowledge, knowledge that, after all, benefits us all.[18]

In the age of stem cell science, it is more important than ever that we broadly agree on the principles and priorities that should drive research. If we can agree, for example, that the patients who, as part of their treatment, donate biological material to research should have a say in how that material is used, then we need to ask what is required to give members of the public a voice in setting research agendas.

Most people don't hold the pre-existing knowledge of experts on the ethical and policy issues surrounding the use of biological materials. This makes pre-framed questions by experts, like those posed to the Lacks family, coercive. First, people need to be informed, they need to have an opportunity to state their hopes for the future of research, to ask questions, voice concerns; they need to be presented with the scope of possibilities, including those that are pre-emptively ruled out by scientists, as well as the ethical challenges associated with them. These discussions need to be conducted in spaces that are inclusive and using language that is accessible. Serious scientific effort needs to go into developing the technologies of participation in science, especially where it is difficult, because resistance marks the points at which this kind of interaction is most lacking, and so points to the groups of people who have had the least say, although they may make the biggest biological contributions to stem cell research.

A question of choice

In 2008, the pharmaceutical company Merck launched a new advert to encourage women to take up Gardasil, their HPV vaccine. Women could empower themselves, the confident prototype patients in the video attest, by protecting themselves from 'two types of HPV that cause cervical cancer, and the two types that cause other HPV diseases'.[19] 'I Chose' became the name of the campaign. A familiar echo of saintliness? Like Henrietta Lacks in her portrait, the responsibility for reproduction these women take is framed as a strange hybrid of empowered sacrifice. And this comes to her as naturally as motherhood.

The predominant question I have asked throughout this chapter is: to what extent can women be said to have a choice about the way their biological material is used? Choices between options or asking for permission don't quite cut it when these decisions are framed as moral obligations or when their investment is discarded as a donation in a system that still demands that women contribute to society in the narrow way it allows – that is, reproductively. Here we might again question how empowered the women in the Merck advert really are when their contributions aren't valued but rather expected.

While women carry the burden of responsibility for HPV screening, as they do for contraception and sexual health in heterosexual partnerships, they also reap the benefits of early detection, as well as the opportunity to get a vaccine for a disease that also affects men. The case of HPV crystalises the consequence of a medicine and science that does not interrogate how gender bias shapes its discoveries and, importantly, also their implementation. A medicine that is all about cutting-edge advance and less about implementation might benefit the careers of a few male scientists, but, ultimately, it hurts us all. As we have already seen in this book, a medicine that is blind to its gendered assumptions will also be blind to its absences. Men, in the advertisement, are invisible, along with any mention of sexual transmission of HPV. They are not responsible for HPV prevention, but this comes at a cost to their health.*

Perhaps, what we really need to ask is: how empowered are we (all) as a society, when the way medicine and science are sacrifices health and truth in order to prop up a set of narrow assumptions about who we are, and the roles we should play?

In the age of stem cell research, as cells flow between fields and across the world, it is clearer than ever that we are all connected through medicine and science – and so we all stand to benefit or be harmed by the work scientists and researchers do. Shifting the balance in favour of that existential divide starts with giving people a choice. Yet a real choice depends on information, on understanding the scope of possibilities.

When experts hold the power to determine the scope of what is medically important or scientifically interesting, talk of

---

* Merck has since revised its advertising strategy to include both genders. Yet, to this day, in the US, most direct-to-consumer advertisements for the vaccine are generally restricted to women's magazines, targeting mothers with adolescents, in particular.

consensus by policy organisations and medical institutions is disingenuous. Their discussions do little to redress the balance in a carnivorous world that feeds some bodies to others. To the list of unanswered scientific questions, we need to add this one: how can we give more people choice in medical and scientific decision making?

Chapter 10

Egg and Sperm

Just as we are finding new ways to read biology, we must also consider rewriting the biological stories we thought we already knew. Yet if there's one story we surely don't need to reconsider, it's this one: egg meets sperm. The story of how an egg, containing half the DNA required to make a human, merges with a sperm, containing the other half, and in this seminal moment in a human life, triggers a process of development that will continue until a woman delivers a child. It's a tale as old as time.

We learn this story young. The protagonist is usually the sperm. Tales of great races, sperm cells defying the odds in their quest to reach the egg. Often, the sperm and egg are personified, to make the story more entertaining to children. The valiant knight rescuing the helpless maiden. But cells aren't people. And the traits we associate with cells affect our understanding of the scientific process – and with it, of men and women too.

In 1991, the anthropologist Emily Martin decided to investigate accounts of fertilisation. She published her findings in her now cult article: 'The Egg and the Sperm: How Science Has Constructed a Romance Based on Stereotypical Male-Female Roles.'[1] Martin examined a range of the most common textbooks used in classes for medical students over the course of several years, analysing their language use. What she found was that the childhood stories about adventuring sperm had wriggled their way into the science.

The depictions of the egg and sperm rely on – and reflect – stereotypes central to our cultural definitions of male and female. These stereotypes imply not only that female biological processes are less worthy than their male counterparts but, as is the trend across medicine, also that women are less worthy than men. Sperm, the language of the textbooks suggested, are produced at an astounding rate, whereas a woman is born with only a finite number of eggs, waiting passively to be used at any time. The sperm are adventurers, braving hostile environments to accomplish their mission. Yet the egg is 'rescued' by the sperm, saved from its fate of being flushed away in menstruation, *wasted*.

This story is just one example of the surprising, pervasive and subtle subliminal messages women receive about their bodies. Along with the choices in textbooks and children's books about how egg and sperm are depicted, are choices made as to what is not depicted? Where does this adventure play out? Where is the princess's castle? What treacherous terrain must the sperm face? It is, of course, the woman's body.

While as we have seen women's bodies have historically, *relentlessly*, been reduced to their reproductive capacity in medicine, women themselves seem to be absent from scientific accounts. It is another narrative function that erases women from the scientific picture, but also gives the sense that their biology is separate from them. That they are passive carriers of a mysterious world within themselves, that should be controlled and monitored by scientists, but not explained to women

– and definitely not investigated in order to benefit women. The magical mystery of fertilisation has always been about babies, a quasi-religious moment within science, nestled deep inside the female body.

A changing landscape

The invisibility of a woman's insides was for a long time more than a cultural belief, but also a scientific limitation. For humans, fertilisation happens out of sight, inside the female uterus, posing a big barrier to understanding how the earliest stages of life emerged. That is until 1978, when a new technique promised to change this. In vitro fertilisation allowed scientists to mimic the process of egg-meets-sperm in a petri dish. In a lab. Thus the goings on within the female uterus were impenetrable no longer.

If there was ever a watershed moment that would change how women were viewed in medicine, surely it would be the moment that the seat of her mystery was turned inside out, her interiority now a movie for anyone to watch in curious wonder. Would this be the end of the scientific containment of a woman within herself? And yet over a decade later, in 1991, the self-same messages about active sperm and passive eggs were still being taught at universities – and they prevail in much of literature today – colouring what most of us know about reproduction.

The possibility of moving baby-making from the womb to the lab raised the hope that women would also move from the margins to the centre of thorough scientific investigation. IVF was undeniably cutting edge, and so presented the possibility that scientists would take reproduction seriously as a high-tech and scientifically prestigious line of inquiry; that this domain, so long side-lined along with women and their supposedly mysterious insides, would finally move to the centre. It should by all rights have been the beginning of scientists getting to know women on their own terms. Yet, it wasn't.

The story of the IVF pioneers has been widely told. It has lent itself especially to cinematic retelling – the striking view down the microscope of two cells meeting; the process of retrieving an egg from the woman's ovaries; the scientist's hand driving the action.

The first baby to be born using this technique was Louise Brown, on 25 July 1978. The story of the 'miracle baby' was reported internationally. Especially in England, where she was born. Newspapers vied for photos of the newborn with her parents. This enthusiastic media response probably came as a relief to the two pioneers behind the new technique. Robert Edwards and Patrick Steptoe had been under pressure from newspapers to allow scrutiny of their work. What they were doing was, after all, not just cutting-edge but very much out there, in barely traversed territory. They were making the leap from a technique only used successfully on animals to humans. The consequences of this kind of tinkering in a process previously hidden from sight on the further development of a human baby were unknown and this was controversial. It divided the scientific community and made many members of the public wary that scientists had finally gone too far, were sacrificing potential lives in their hunger for scientific knowledge.

Edwards and Steptoe persevered for various reasons, undoubtedly including advancing scientific understanding. The reason most cited to the public, however, was the benefit

IVF would offer to couples struggling to conceive. It allowed Lesley and John Brown to overcome the barrier of Lesley's blocked fallopian tubes (meaning that the egg and sperm could not meet in Lesley's body), allowing her to get pregnant after over nine years of trying unsuccessfully to conceive naturally. Louise turned out to be a perfectly healthy baby and, as it turns out, over forty years later, a healthy adult too.

Given the controversy around their work, the research pair agreed to a deal with Associated Newspapers. They and the parents also allowed the government's Central Office of Information to film Louise's birth, which was broadcast on national television. They also formed a close relationship with the journalist Peter Williams, who produced a documentary about Louise that aired when she was just six weeks old on ITV called *To Mrs Brown . . . A Daughter*. The documentary showed in detail just how IVF worked. For the vast majority of its viewers this would have been the first time they saw the moment of fertilisation at all, let alone in a petri dish. And their guide was Robert Edwards, filmed in his laboratory by Williams.

To perform IVF, scientists monitor and simulate a woman's ovulation to remove an egg from her ovaries, then place this in liquid, a 'culture medium', with a sperm cell. The fertilised egg is left to divide for several days, before it is placed into a woman's uterus with the intention that it will implant itself in the lining to establish a pregnancy. In the documentary, viewers watch Edwards as he examines the contents of his 'collecting chamber' of eggs under the microscope, how he removes an egg and places it in the culture medium in the petri dish. The climax of the conception story is, of course, fertilisation. A sperm heroically arriving to save his swooning damsel in distress. And here, a dramatic close-up shows how Edwards holds the egg in a pipette ready for the decisive moment. Only where are the sperm vying for entry? The familiar romance isn't what begins to unfold. The egg is the one doing the moving instead. Against all we thought was natural, it moves towards the sperm. 'In she goes,' Edwards says, as he releases the egg from the pipette. 'Here,' says Williams' voiceover, 'is the act of in vitro fertilisation; the moment of conception outside the human body.'

There we have it. Reproduction post-IVF. A scientifically exacting, hyper-visible performance that moved from the mysterious depths of the womb into the public eye. New protagonists overlapping with the old – egg and sperm still involved, but now another key player, in the form of the scientist's hand. The scientist was now intimately involved in a process, fertilisation, that had previously been played out ever so discretely in bedrooms around the world, and ever so silently inside the woman's reproductive system.

In the post-IVF era, women can turn to scientists for assistance. Reproduction no longer only happens in private, but in labs too. IVF has made reproduction a serious area of scientific inquiry. It has gone some way in tackling the view that female reproductive biology is impenetrable to science, and therefore not serviceable by medical care. With this scientific insight, social views have also started to shift. As we'll see, IVF makes it possible for men and women in different kinds of relationships to have biological children too, or for women to do so using sperm donors, or at an older age. These technical possibilities help provide alternatives for a framework where women are solely responsible for reproduction, and are defined by their reproductive capacities. IVF and other reproductive technologies can help facilitate a shift in gender roles with implications that go beyond reproduction. IVF brings the hope that a new era in science could be a new era for the treatment of women, and of the valuing of reproduction and childbearing in medicine and society too.

On a cellular level, IVF allows us to revisit the conception story we thought we knew, revealing that the 'personalities' of egg and sperm have long been misrepresented. It is, for example, not necessarily the first sperm to arrive that fertilises the egg – it takes much more than one to accomplish the job. This is far from a traditional romance. Moreover, the egg is not simply passively 'penetrated' by the sperm.

In 2016, researchers at Berkeley found that the egg, sensing sperm nearby, sends out a wave of progesterone which activates a receptor on a sperm's tail, giving it a 'power kick', a boost to make it swim faster as it covers that last harrowing distance.[2] This shower of progesterone also helps the tail of the sperm break through the egg's protective coating. Without this boost, fertilisation won't happen. Further research, conducted in 2020 by researchers at the University of Manchester and Stockholm University Sweden, has even suggested that the egg 'chooses' the best quality sperm.[3] The fluid that surrounds the egg when it is released from the ovaries acts as chemical attractant to the sperm, and contains chemical signals that likely draw in sperm that is more genetically compatible. In other words? The egg plays an essential, *active* role in conception.

This research also suggests another fallacy that accompanies the depiction of sperm – namely, that they are active adventurers. The mechanism between egg and sperm required to spur them along suggests that sperm don't have the agency or

consciousness required to justify their role as the story's protagonist. Fertilisation is an interaction. Sperm cells move randomly,
without clear direction or intention. From the perspective of
sperm, it is chance – compounded by their prolific numbers
– that ensures that every once in a while, they reach an egg,
while the egg asserts an arguably greater influence on the
outcome. Even in this new rendition of a romance, with an
active egg, we must be wary of anthropomorphising these cells
– of attributing human characteristics to them – as these are
the loaded ideas that, as we have seen, tend to prejudice
research. If we do insist on anthropomorphising, however,
then we would have to concede that sperm present the most
unreliable, unconscious knights in shining armour – and that
the egg never needed rescuing at all.

The possibility of watching and manipulating cells outside
of the woman's body has allowed scientists to challenge assumptions about egg and sperm, although as the forty-year lag
between Louise Brown's birth and these new findings about
sperm suggests, this has been a slow process. Views of male and
female roles in courtship are so entrenched that scientists don't
see what they don't know. These assumptions are like water to
fish or sperm, if we ourselves also choose to stick to that
misguided analogy – they are ubiquitous, part of the fabric of
our world. It takes more than new laboratory techniques
of visualisation to bring these to light. It requires perspective.

The framing of the conception story, even post-IVF,
remained resolutely myopic. The frame of the petri dish
marked the limits of the designated territory on their map.
The scientists studied these cells in a vacuum. The image of
these cells handled by a scientist became iconic for the break-
through possibilities IVF held for creating life in the lab. What

we didn't see in these images though, what none of them showed, was the woman's body.

While fertilisation through IVF was now possible in a lab, it was still women who carried these fertilised egg cells to term. Indeed, while the scientist's hand may have been introduced into their revised conception story, the pioneers behind IVF had no interest in introducing the mother as an active character. As they talked people through the technique on television, they were careful to limit the bounds of their narrative, to insist that this was still the cosy, domestic story they all knew and shared, as the sociologist Katie Dow has documented,[4] all the while using comforting, familiar language, lulling the viewers into a new bedtime conception story. Edwards describes placing the egg in the culture medium as putting it 'home', reassures the viewer that the egg is now 'safe'. When he looks at it under the microscope, he coos that it is 'a lovely egg, a very nice egg indeed'. Despite the futuristic setting of the lab, the scientist's gloved hand guiding the process, it is a bizarrely domestic scene. And, for Edwards and Steptoe, this framing of their narrative was necessary in order to reassure a largely conservative British public that IVF would fit into their idea of the nuclear family. It was accordingly framed as a technique that would help infertile couples in traditional, heterosexual relationships, and was thus used to reinforce a familiar story, to further entrench the role of women as silent baby-carriers. In other words, IVF in its original framing was about making babies and consolidating families, rather than about expanding the options or improving the care available to women.

IVF may have moved fertilisation out of the uterus, but, to this day, the female body is still heavily involved in the process. The procedure is deeply invasive. It requires that women endure a process of stimulation, egg retrieval, insemination, embryo culture and transfer. Stimulation involves receiving fertility drugs, often injections, containing hormones to increase the number of eggs the patient's body produces. Besides the various physiological and emotional effects of these drugs, doctors perform regular blood tests and scans to monitor the production of eggs until they are ready to retrieve. Egg retrieval is a surgical procedure requiring anaesthesia. Transfer involves inserting a thin tube containing the embryo, called a catheter, into the vagina, past the cervix and into the uterus, where it is released. These techniques have not been adequately developed or reconsidered in the decades since Louise Brown was born because the aim was simply to retrieve eggs and achieve conception. The wellbeing of the woman only mattered insofar as it guaranteed the wellbeing of the embryo. Sound familiar?

The chances of complications are, in fact, higher for IVF pregnancies: multiple pregnancies, which in turn might lead to premature birth, miscarriage, ectopic pregnancy (when the eggs implant outside the uterus), bleeding, infection or damage to the bowels or bladder and ovarian hyperstimulation syndrome (OHSS). That is an exaggerated response to excess hormones that causes the ovaries to swell and become painful that can, in the worst cases, be fatal. All this, along with the emotional strain that comes with managing expectations in a procedure that is still likely not to result in pregnancy at all.

Infertility in a twenty-first century context

Over forty years after its first success, IVF remains an experimental technique. The success rate averages at around 20% per monthly cycle for women in the UK and the US, and this decreases with age. While the technique is offered widely, it is far from the fail-safe path to pregnancy to which many clinics attest – many charging hefty fees. Women's invisibility from the IVF picture, shown to the public in the news and in science articles to this day, is mirrored in this disregard in the IVF industry for the impact of the technique on the female body. Once again, science needs to turn to its blind spots, to continue to develop its methods to respond to the needs of the people it purports to serve. The invention of a new technique or the discovery of a new phenomenon can never be the end of the scientific story.

In comparison to this demanding regime in female bodies, the procedure performed on the male body is small. For insemination, a male donor or partner will be required to produce a semen sample, which a technician will combine with the egg in a petri dish and will monitor while it divides and grows until it is ready to implant. While the emotional burden for the non-carrying partners involved in IVF should not be under-estimated and, indeed, is only just opening up as an area that needs to be more deliberately addressed, the point is that there are possible routes to achieving pregnancy that are less invasive for the woman. These target the sperm instead, and have not been considered because of an inability to think outside of our familiar conception stories – the ones in which female bodies are solely responsible for childbirth. The design of the IVF process has continued to mimic this entrenched, outdated division of labour, rather than seizing the creative opportunities technological assistance offers to reimagine how men and women could share responsibility for reproduction.

So how could we reimagine the role of men in IVF?

Given the cultural merging of women with reproduction, fertility is one of the few areas in which research on male biology lags behind. Some have pointed to the use of intracytoplasmic sperm injection (ICSI) as an explanation for the neglect of specific studies on sperm functioning in the process of fertilisation. First performed successfully in a clinical setting in 1990, ICSI involves the injection of a single sperm directly into a mature egg to assist in fertilisation, especially when sperm seems to be at fault. This rather crude mechanical method has offered a work-around when sperm does not seem to function normally, but in doing so has also stymied research into the underlying causes of these deficiencies, and so a lack of understanding of male infertility or the development of non-invasive therapeutic techniques that target the male patient. There are many genetic and epigenetic defects involved in the production of sperm that have yet to be explored, especially the effects of lifestyle factors such as smoking, age and obesity on sperm DNA. Tackling these lifestyle factors may offer an alternative to ICSI, and also its associated risks, which include increased incidence of miscarriage, risks for the health of the offspring and even passing infertility on to future generations.

Perhaps the failure to look beyond ICSI is itself the consequence of lingering ideas about women in natural conception as the passive receptacles of invasive procedures – coupled with the historically incorrect yet incredibly pervasive idea that fertility problems come from women. New technologies in themselves will not change if scientists and medical professionals refuse to consider how these outdated ideas will frame what they choose to see.

Research on sperm biology is one area which, as well as

increasing knowledge of male infertility and finding new treatments to optimise natural conception, will offer new options for those who wish to conceive before turning to methods for assisted conception like IVF. Identifying new sperm components that can be pharmacologically or otherwise corrected may prove less invasive (and less expensive) than fertility treatment. In cases where the cause of infertility is uncertain, examining sperm might point to the man as the main contributor to the couple's infertility, so that he might be the primary patient to be treated. As long as there is no research into the role of sperm in fertility, however, the female will often be treated as the patient when it's a male disease.

The legacy of IVF is anything but straightforward. Old ideas about gender continue to linger as sticky visitations that shape everything we know. But, like a moiré pattern, new ideas have also begun to shine through. The effect can be disorientating. For example, when a lesbian couple decides to use IVF to conceive a child using donated sperm, they are able to be sure they are both genetically related to the child by using the mitochondria from one mother (which contains small amounts of her DNA) and inserting it into an egg from the other mother.

Here we have a retelling of the conception story in which a non-heterosexual couple is able to mimic the merging of DNA we see at fertilisation between egg and sperm. You could argue that in imitating the traditional story, they reinforce ideas about a man and a woman coming together to produce a child, but they have also changed it because they have reproduced the story with a difference – one in which a non-heterosexual couple, with or without a surrogate, representing a social arrangement that diverges from the nuclear family, have made particular choices, using the helping hand of a scientist, to establish the kind of family they want. This will come with a different division of mothering tasks – starting with the idea that it is a woman in a heterosexual relationship who is responsible for fertility, conception, childbearing and birth – that will demand that medical practitioners pay heed to these differences, as will society at large, changing their ideas of what a woman is, can be and should do.

Pioneering moments are more complicated than the images in the news or in science make them out to be. They don't end where the frame does, or at least, there are forces at work that set those frames and begin to tug and pull at those frames, imploring scientists to go further, to see something new. Pioneering isn't just done by scientists; it is done by the people who take up these techniques and reinvent them as they make them their own. Slowly, we learn to look further, to go further, and expand the frame.

PART 3

Future Bodies

Change is born in the imagination. For any change to happen, we need to be able to imagine it first, and this is no less true for science. So far, we've worked hard to break with past narratives, to find new visions of a science and a medicine that responds to the needs of all bodies. We've followed unheard voices, expanded our narrative, and have asked scientists to take up new perspectives. Another place to look for a vision of a new science is the cutting-edge of technology – the brand-new innovations, or those on the verge of being implemented. As I've argued throughout this book, high-tech interventions aren't always necessary to shift care and attention to the problems that matter to women. Some of them, however, are excellent tools for the imagination. The technologies we'll see exist on a tantalising boundary between what is and what could be. They gesture to a new future. All we have to do is pick them up.

The most exciting technological possibilities in medicine for women are those we can use to subvert the gendered ideas that have long marked the limits of what can be known about our bodies. These inventions engage with the process of reproduction – diagnostic tampons, 3D clitorises, artificial wombs and endometrium models. Yet they also straddle a host of other disciplines. What is so promising about many of the new interventions in reproduction today is that they require inter-disciplinary collaborations, forcing scientists and medical professionals to draw connections across disciplines, allowing them to tackle questions that extend beyond their traditional purviews, beyond the limits of the questions we associate with reproduction, and so also beyond traditional views of a woman's reproductive function. Suddenly, a womb can teach us about immunology, for example. This process implicitly begins to tackle restrictive, gendered thinking in medicine, potentially reshaping its tools around the much broader array of questions that matter to women and their health.

In other cases, the challenge to gendered thinking is more explicit. Artificial wombs, for example, force scientists to revisit assumptions about the female body in gestation, so closely tied to naturalised ideas about motherhood. In these cases, questioning restrictive, gendered ideas is necessary in the development of safe and effective technologies, let alone in decisions about how we implement them as a society. In all these examples, there are opportunities but also a plethora of ways in which these tools can be co-opted by practitioners of the well-established, male-centric science to perpetuate harmful gendered thinking and restrict women's freedoms, harm their health and inhibit scientific progress. We have to be wary of the misuse of these exciting new tools, at the same time that we have to be boldly optimistic about the possibili-ties we can use them to generate. One thing's for sure, as with the advent of IVF, these technologies prove that reproduction is by no means the backwater of innovative science (as if it ever was) but its most exciting and generative frontier, because its technological possibilities open our eyes to new visions of social progress.

How helpful these technological interventions can be will depend on how we use them. Like all the science we have seen, these tools are shaped by the culture that holds them, but they also hold a glimpse of something more. All the examples are uncanny familiar unfamiliars, reinventions of objects and organs whose meaning had become naturalised in a patriarchal medical system. Now they look different, and serve a different purpose. Their artificial freakishness demands that we look anew at the 'natural' womanhood we thought we knew, and follow them, imaginations first, into a future in which technology aids social progress.

Chapter 11

Femtech

I'd heard the horror stories.

Forgotten tampons.

Our teacher in sex education class had warned us about the dangers . . .

Potentially life-threatening.

Floating around in a uterus like some lonely astronaut, left in there long enough, they could go septic.

Nonetheless, something had driven me that mid-morning in my early teens, during my free hour before History class, to give tampons a go. It wasn't for lack of alternatives lying around the house. Usually, I would have gone for one of the thick pads Mum kept in the cupboard under the sink. I found them reassuringly infantilising, the way they mimicked a nappy, a cushy mattress swelling up between my legs, reminding me that I was supported, safe. Today, however, I'd made a conscious decision to leave the comfort of visible support structures behind. I'd decided I wanted to be part of the Club.

My mum's tampons, like my mum herself, weren't as cool as the ones many of my classmates had. She'd clearly opted for the cheapest brand. Just a bland collection of clinical, white cotton buds. Practical. No applicators, no extravagant floral wrapping, no scents or girl-power slogans. Very mum. I opened the box and picked up one of the – what suddenly struck me was sort of bullet-shaped – tampons. I fiddled around with the plastic, trying not to rip any of the compact cotton enclosed inside. I knew how they worked. I'd seen them in action, when my brother's friend had dunked about ten in water before hanging them on the Christmas tree as a joke. I'd stared wide-eyed at the enormity of the white sponges, trying to imagine how something that size could possibly fit inside the worm-hole between my legs. Now, I forced myself to suppress the thought that this was a ticking time-bomb. This innocent-looking cotton bud had the propensity to expand, rising inside me like bread. There seemed to me a mechanistic incompati-bility between my vagina and this tampon.

I leaned over to try to get a better view of what I was doing, watched my hands as they held the white thing awkwardly in a pincer-like grip. I was terrified that I'd stick it up the wrong hole. What exactly I imagined would happen if I did, I wasn't sure, but the region between my legs seemed like an ominous landscape. When I'd finally checked to make sure it was the *lower one, definitely the lower one,* I slowly pressed the surpris-ingly solid thing inside of me. This is natural, I told myself. This is what women do. My body was a machine, this tampon, a predetermined screw.

My vagina, though, disagreed. My muscles clenched as I pushed harder, trying to expel the foreign entity I'd intro-duced. Ignoring the stinging in my pelvic floor as I pushed through the discomfort, my chest fluttered, heart rate soared. I could feel the panic rising, then the tampon passed some kind of a ridge, popping as if I'd opened a celebratory bottle. As if.

White light.

Darkness.

I woke up with my cheek against the cold tiles of the bathroom floor, jeans around my ankles and a strange fuzzy feeling between my legs. Still light-headed, I sat up and grasped desperately for the string, tugging at it, first gently, then, when nothing happened, with more force, until the rough cotton edged slowly, reluctantly out. It was still the same size. No exponential rising, and just a faint tint of pink at the tip. I tossed it in the bin, then checked my phone. I was late. I grabbed a pad from my bag and stuck it to my knickers. I looked at it, defeated and at the same time, at some level, somehow feeling reaffirmed. I'd been doing what was right to me all along. I ran to school and told the teacher I'd lost track of time.

To me, the tampon was always a sub-optimal solution to the supposed problem that is menstruation. The very premise of the thing plugging up a hole seems crass, seems to defy what a period is – flow.

The founders of NextGen Jane agree.

Tampon science

To Ridhi Tariyal and Stephen Gire of NextGen Jane, the tampon isn't the endpoint, the plug in a conversation about what women feel and need, but the very beginning, opening up new fertile terrain to explore on the road to expanding the options to *all* bodies in medicine. And so, the humble tampon takes flight. The two bioengineers have reclaimed the tampon as a diagnostic tool, one that can point to conditions specific to people who menstruate, such as endometriosis. Using the menstrual blood squeezed from used tampons, they hope to find early markers of endometriosis and eventually cervical cancer and various other disorders.

I described in the very opening of the book, my horror at the casual way in which my gynaecologist suggested inserting a camera into my pelvic cavity through a surgical incision. This is a common procedure currently required to diagnose women with endometriosis, to look for endometrial cells in places other than the lining of the uterus, which characterise the disease. It requires an anaesthetic, is never risk-free and leaves scarring. If abnormal cells are found, these can be removed, but the average woman diagnosed with endometriosis will have had the disease for over a decade, along with all the accompanying pain.

NextGen Jane is all about prevention. Once they have conducted sufficient clinical trials to establish the diagnostic efficacy of menstrual blood, they hope their tampon will allow doctors to identify endometriosis ahead of time. Their current patent is simply for a device that wrings out menstrual blood, but this tool is just the beginning, a so-called 'platform technology' that will allow them to build on the current possibilities, to diagnose other conditions and, ultimately, to implement the coveted lifespan-approach to medicine we so desperately need.

The company is also focused on the preventative care that is the aspiration of many of the most forward-thinking gynae-cologists and obstetricians mentioned in the opening chapters of this book. Indeed, NextGen Jane's key tenet is early detec-tion technologies; treatment options are good; avoiding the need for them is even better. This means reframing diagnosis as a one-off event, and instead basing it on a series of observa-tions made throughout a person's life. What NextGen Jane are advocating is the kind of life-course approach to medical care that, for a long time, we could scarcely even dream of.

Only now that life-course approach begins to resemble the sexy science that previously left women in the dust. High-tech science, of course, was never inherently problematic, only how it was used. Modern technology can bring us high-tech solutions to gender bias in medicine – provided that we understand that technology will only ever be a tool in that process, never in and of itself a silver bullet solution.

The technologised tampon is part of a new medical story, a story with a different pace, and a different kind of teleology – the tampon is the beginning, diagnosis isn't the climax, only the framework for an ongoing interaction between the patient and the medical options available to them. Reorganising the medical narrative is not easy – as we have seen, it meets bureaucratic and ideological resistance along the way in a culture attached to the power structures that put male bodies at the centre, on top, in power. Yet we have also seen how new stories sneak in when they are told by people on the margins, people straddling fields and disciplines, reproducing the familiar images of hearts or egg and sperm or female genitals with a tweak; changes that reveal how our concepts are mutable. Showing us that there is more to what we thought we knew. This tampon is another such sly little package, smuggling in a host of new possibilities, expanding and rising – this time not inside the body of a muted girl, and instead disrupting a field with its ability to absorb much more than menstrual blood, but a several cutting-edge fields of science too.

NextGen Jane forms part of a wave of new women's health products dubbed 'femtech', in 2016, by the Danish entrepreneur Ida Tin, the CEO of Clue, a mobile menstrual health app created by Berlin-based BioWink GmbH, a company she co-founded in 2013. In just another example of the labour of care women in top professions continue to perform, Tin coined the term to mitigate men's discomfort with discussing issues like incontinence and menstruation. This way, as Tin explained during a 2018 Geekettes panel: '. . . investors can say, "I have four FemTech companies in my portfolio" instead of "I have a company for women peeing in their pants." That's hard for a male investor to say.'[1]

Tin frames the need to make men 'comfortable' discussing technology that serves to increase women's wellbeing as a pragmatic choice. Part of me admires her for her by any means approach to sneaking important women's health issues into an industry dominated by men; for working within the system to achieve her goals. Another part of me is furious that this is necessary. The risk is that the appeasing power of the term will do more than sneak products into investors' portfolios, that it perpetuates the gendered assumptions by framing the host of products targeted at women in terms that undermine their disruptive presence to put male investors at ease.

When people talk about femtech now, they are referring to a subset of medical technology products and services, not simply marketed to women but addressing issues historically and conventionally associated with the reproductive health of cisgender women. In recent years, Silicon Valley has brought to market a wide array of products and services addressing issues like contraception and fertility, pregnancy and post-pregnancy, breastfeeding, menstruation and period care, pelvic health, menopause, hormonal disorders (e.g. polycystic ovary syndrome) and sexual wellness.

Women can now purchase menstrual cycle tracking apps and gadgets ('Fitbit for your period'); organic, chemical-free, reusable and home-delivered feminine hygiene products;

at-home fertility tests; urinary tract infection-preventing pink lemonade powder; apps that deliver birth control and antibiotics (for the UTIs that can't be prevented). The femtech business may be booming – Frost & Sullivan, a market research firm, predicts that femtech will be a $50 billion industry by 2025 – yet women's healthcare, as attested by the firm, 'remains largely confined to reproductive matters'.[2] Moreover, when compared to The Digital Health industry as a whole, predicted by some to reach somewhere between $500 and $600 billion in that same year,[3] it is clear that women continue to represent a subsidiary, if growing, branch of healthtech, as much as they are in medicine.

In the media, femtech is often lauded as an empowering, equalising industry, giving female entrepreneurs, designers and patients the opportunity to balance the scales in healthcare provision through their inclusion in a tech industry as male-dominated as science. Yet the name of the sector itself already reveals the extent to which old-fashioned mores, as well as old-fashioned power structures, restrict innovation to the spheres traditionally associated with cisgender women – often in very uncreative ways.

Within femtech, for example, smartphone apps that are mainly marketed as providing 'fertility awareness' are among the most popular health-tracking technologies in high-income countries and are gaining popularity around the world. These apps help identify the 'fertile window' within the menstrual cycle when conception is most likely, based on a wide range of personal information, such as users' mood, sexual and physical activity, bodily signs, symptoms and dimensions. In the UK, around a third of cisgender women using fertility awareness apps are doing so to support conception.[4] As for the other two-thirds, these women might be using them for a host of other reasons, including but not limited to predicting periods and managing symptoms like pain or mood fluctuations or preventing pregnancy. Even within the scope of fertility, these apps often misrepresent what they might mean to women, let alone the aspects of health and sex that matter to women that are completely disregarded. While journalists claim these apps offer women greater bodily autonomy and even 'revolutionise birth control',[5] they often reinforce normative gendered assumptions – the apps that are geared towards monitoring sexual pleasure and performance are almost exclusively aimed at men, while those tracking fertility, pregnancy and planned parenting are aimed at women,[6] with little consideration for sexual and gender diversity.

In 2015, Maggie Delano, now Assistant Professor of Engineering at Swarthmore College, Pennsylvania, was one of the first to voice these criticisms.[7] Delano describes how, as a queer woman with irregular periods who is not interested in having children, she felt erased by the apps she tried, diminished by the monotonous heteronormative assumptions embedded within the apps that relentlessly categorised women as either wanting babies or not wanting babies. Without any provision for a woman's sexual desires. No care for the fact that at least two-thirds of an app's users, at any given time, might be solely interested in tracking their symptoms in order to better manage them or that many more women are interested in contraception than conception.

Since 2015, the backlash against femtech has become more widespread, with others in the media echoing Delano's observations,[8] arguing that femtech pigeonholes women's health[9] and reduces women to reproductive biological functions while simultaneously excluding non-binary and trans users.[10] In this conflicted space, the founders of NextGen Jane launched their brand, a space where mentors continually recommended that instead of 'menstrual blood', they used the 'more scientific' (read less overtly female-centric) 'female substrate'.[11] 'We wish we could go out there and say we just want to diagnose women's diseases,' Tariyal said in one interview. But investors would ask her: 'Where's the money in that?'[12]

This choice wasn't strategic or disingenuous, and this is also not the point I am making. Fertility is a worthy cause – I am in no way trying to diminish it. Tariyal even started her fertility-centred project in 2013 on a fellowship at Harvard Business School designed to encourage graduates to start new life sciences companies, in an effort, again, to focus on putting women's needs at the centre of treatment. And, indeed, there is much work to be done in this arena still. But, as has been the argument throughout this book, this category has subsumed all areas of women's health. It has stifled research that would blur the lines between the neatly delineated fields and bodily systems that scientists have become invested in. In the case of NextGen Jane, the early motivations were intimately entwined with Tariyal's own fertility concerns. At the time of her fellowship, she was thirty-three and knew she wanted children eventually, but she wasn't ready yet. She asked her doctor at the time if she could wait five more years before she tried. She wanted to do a blood test called an anti-Müllerian hormone (or AMH) test that would approximate the number of viable eggs she had. But her doctor didn't see the need and wouldn't order it for her, then told her instead that the best test she was going to get was to try to get pregnant and see if it worked.

So began the early venturing into femtech 'proper'. Partnering with Gire, Tariyal set out to design assays, methods to measure proteins that would let her determine whether AMH and other hormones could be detected in menstrual blood, instead of blood drawn from veins, so that women wouldn't have to see a doctor to get tested, and they could simply do the tests from home. Tariyal performed tests that looked at three types of samples – venous blood, blood from a pinprick to the skin and menstrual blood – to see where they overlapped. To her disappointment, she found that AMH levels are consistently lower in menstrual blood than they are in venous blood, making it an ineffective fertility test. Yet testing the different blood types had revealed that menstrual blood contained something that was different but useful – namely, very clear genomic signals, that is, genes that are expressed differently in menstrual blood compared to venous blood. She found some 800 of these genes. Menstrual 'effluence' contains not only blood but also endometrial lining, and some cervical and vaginal cells as well. These qualities meant that, according to Tariyal, it was like 'getting a natural biopsy from your body'.[13]

A natural biopsy.

This oxymoronic phrase is quoted across the media coverage of NextGen Jane's promising new technique. It's a contradiction in terms because it describes a method in the context of a highly technologised and interventional procedure as 'natural'.

A biopsy is taken for analysis by scientists; it is a concept that describes an already scientific procedure. It is, of course, anything but 'unassisted by science' – if that's what we mean by 'natural'. But that's the very genius and the point of NextGen Jane's approach – that it challenges what we imagine to be natural biology, because it opens up new potentialities – the potential as a diagnostic tool for all sorts of diseases – to the familiar, defining aspects of female biology we thought we knew.

Though genomic analysis wasn't her goal, when Tariyal stumbled across this possibility, she let her findings guide her. The tampon is Tariyal's unintended chimera – piggybacking on femtech's myopic focus on fertility (because what is menstruation if not simply a mark of fertility . . .?) and then using technology to demonstrate that fluids and organs associated with reproduction can be part of other diagnostic systems, can be multidimensional and can bear relevance to the health of all other parts of the body. In doing so, NextGen Jane has managed to redefine the relationship between women and medicine.

Research programmes like NextGen Jane turn femtech, just like the tampon, into an exploratory space that doesn't define a single version of woman by her biology, but tests and stretches this category to see how far it will go by introducing new technology into the mix. The so-called 'Smart Tampon' is a strategic step towards including women in the purview of mainstream medicine, but it is just one step. The ultimate goal will be to draw on the findings it gives us to reveal that the gynaecological issues so long considered to mark the limits of the difference of female bodies to men cannot be understood unless we understand their relationship to all of the body's systems. Femtech as a subfield will no longer be distinguishable from other medtech or healthtech companies because 'female' will describe a new body of integrated systems – of reproductive systems and immune systems and genomic systems configured in such a way that gender will not tell us anything close to everything we want to know. The knowledge gained from the investigations on the border of gynaecology and other disciplines will reveal new dimensions of the bodily systems we thought we knew, and these will be relevant to male bodies and all bodies. In time, new disciplines will form around these intersections, undoing the assumptions we have made about gender as the thing that answers our questions. Instead, it will be the starting point: a gender-conscious approach will shape everything we do know.

Menstrual blood, for example, will no longer be defined as reproductive waste but will be treated as a source of genetic information that could be relevant to all humans – a material with purpose (beyond its historic realm of fertility) and value in areas as far ranging as, for example, diagnosing heritable diseases, screening for pelvic inflammation, fibroids, environmental toxins and early cancer. And of course, screening for fertility too.

Reproduction, for female bodies, will be part of the picture, alongside the plethora of other issues that matter to all types of bodies, making the term 'femtech' as obsolete as 'mentech' already is – because tech will cater to everyone.

We'll be looking at a kind of medicine that can harness the body's monthly 'natural biopsy' to monitor health, and not just diagnose disease, a medicine that brings technology and bodies together to unobtrusively provide information that can inform an individual's healthcare decisions. This is ambitious storytelling, this is how we re-engineer a future in a new image – not male, not female, but, potentially, personalised. The most exciting femtech is not the technology that proposes to monitor and regulate female biology, it is the technology that has the power to weave female-specific concerns into the fabric of male-centric science.

When I first turned to tampons it was because I felt I had no choice. I was driven by unarticulated pressures, making the tampon the end to a conversation about my period, about what a period meant. It meant that I continued to carry ideas that my menstruation was somehow tied primarily to my being sexually attractive in the eyes of men, and of the other women onto whom I projected those same ideas. Menstruation was about 'women's issues' which defined and, at the same time, excluded my general health. If this is what being a 'natural' woman means, I don't want to be one. I'd rather have a Smart Tampon designed for a new era in which my period is fertile ground for scientific inquiry that serves my own wellbeing (and that of others like me), in which my body is an important scientific frontier at the heart of an expanding set of choices that sets me and my body free.

Chapter 12

CLITERACY

How do you give women choice? The second wave feminist Betty Dodson had her own answer: 'Better orgasms, better world.' From the early 1970s and right up to her death at ninety-one, in 2020, Dodson taught women – over 7,000 – to achieve orgasm to give them agency over their own bodies and sex lives. For Dodson, this was about more than spreading pleasure, although pleasure was an integral and highly valued part of the project – it was about showing women what independence felt like. When women 'run the fuck', as she so unabashedly put it, men become optional, there not because you need them, only if you want them. The same became true of reproduction – sex was there for pleasure, that of women as much as men, and babies were one possible outcome in the spiral of life. And the same became true for women in any other position in society – it provided a vision of autonomy.

'The most consistent sex will be the love affair you have with yourself,' Dodson wrote in *Sex for One*,[1] a quasi-memoir and how-to guide that has been translated into twenty-five languages since it was first published in 1987. 'Masturbation will get you through childhood, puberty, romance, marriage and divorce, and it will see you through old age.' The bedroom was a model for society – it was about giving women a choice.

As far as it still often feels we have to go in terms of sexual empowerment, that Dodson's statement does not register as nearly as shocking today shows that things have progressed — that there is at least more of a discussion around women's pleasure.

The story of medicine is a history of increasingly advanced techniques being used to solve the problems deemed valuable by men and for male bodies. We've seen repeatedly throughout this book how even when technological options are available, they're often used to consolidate existing prejudices, disguised as conception stories or generalised facts about the human body that only really apply to male systems. We have seen how, as a result, often the answer to addressing research questions that matter to non-male bodies is not necessarily technological innovation but rather using the tools we have and applying them to different problems. Or in some cases, simply organising the delivery of the care we do have differently to respond to the needs of individuals over the course of their lives.

But there are other ways, different scientific ways, in which we can use technology to advance science not just by applying tools to new medical problems but by drawing new participants into the discussions about medicine and the direction it takes. Medical technologies like IVF, we have now seen, are powerful storytelling devices. The images in medicine drive the research in new directions. Yet these often omit important realities. If we acknowledge that medical technologies are storytelling devices, as much as investigatory tools, we can see how giving new people access to these tools changes the narratives we tell in medicine, reframes the questions we ask and drives science in new directions.

Images were central to Dodson's method. After starting her feminist career making erotic art, she began hosting consciousness-raising groups in her Manhattan apartment. This involved what she called a genital 'show-and-tell'. Women gathered naked and Dodson guided them as they looked at each other's vulvas, demonstrating that these come in all shapes, sizes and colours. Only after this did they home in on the clitoris with a vibrator. What a contrast to the dildo-like plethysmograph we saw scientists use in Part 1 of this book, that imposing, foreign, scientific tentacle that forced a reading out of its subjects' bodies in the least arousing of conditions. Dodson was all about giving women control of the technology she offered them – tools meant nothing if you didn't know how to use them.

The clitoris was what women really needed to learn about. A glaring omission from sex education to this day. Only about 20% of women orgasm from vaginal intercourse alone, for the rest, clitoral stimulation is pretty much essential,[2] and so Dodson's method of making women penetrable to themselves became a calling to put the clitoris in the spotlight. With her combined writing and workshopping, she was remarkably influential. Sex educator and activist Carol Queen, who met Betty in the 1980s as part of her doctoral work in sexology, observed: 'Women flocked to her workshops, and some stayed around to develop their own styles of teaching, or activist work, or went back to school so they could be therapists or midwives or whatever style of work that would let them be themselves and make a difference. I'm not sure there's anyone I know of in the sexuality activists of my generation who wasn't inspired (and in many cases egged on) by Betty.'[3] Yet as widespread as this consciousness-raising was, the second wave of openness about female pleasure seemed to have dwindled by 2020.

Goop makes a reappearance here, this time with an episode featuring a ninety-year-old Dodson, as part of the six-part Netflix series Goop Lab. She was there to teach Paltrow the masturbation technique, by this point in its fiftieth year and taught all over the world. The episode surprised viewers, me included, as Paltrow's peppy pseudo-emancipation is stripped back. Dodson, with her no-nonsense attitude, easily punctures through Paltrow's supposedly taboo-breaking, up-beat, school child-like exclamations of the word 'vagina!'. After explaining the vagina is only the birth canal, Dodson adds drily, 'Ya wanna talk about the vulva. That's the clitoris, the inner lips and all that good shit around it.' The conversation then pushes Paltrow to blush when she is made to repeat 'run the fuck'. It does make you wonder whether for all her brazen talk about female genitals, when it comes to empowering herself sexually, she isn't as ballsy as she'd like us to think.

The episode is touching, as Paltrow and her Goop Lab colleagues discuss how they have come to prize looking sexy to others over feeling sexy. Not least Paltrow, who having spent most of her career as an on-screen sex symbol, admits that she is only just beginning to learn how to put her own desires first. Perhaps it comes as no surprise that Goop has done little to further Dodson's efforts to put female experience at the centre, given this revelation.

Just as women seem to have been diminished in contemporary discussions about sex, the clitoris, too, appears to have been demoted from its celebrity status, taking a step back while brighter stars like Paltrow and Goop apparently teach women how to be sexy, rather than feel *sexual*. As recently as 2017, the

French engineer, sociologist and independent researcher Odile Fillod tried her own version of show-and-tell when she produced a 3D-printed model of a clitoris to challenge text-book depictions of female anatomy, and with it persistently misguided ideas about female sexuality. In her independent research on sex and gender issues in biomedical science, Fillod had repeatedly noticed the absence of a correct representation of the clitoris (and even, in some cases, the absence of a mention of the clitoris) in a large number of textbooks supposed to teach what female genital organs look like. She saw this as particularly problematic in the context of sex education, where social norms were linked to this inaccurate biological information. In France, for example, she had noticed that curricula teach 'that boys are more focused on genital sexuality, whereas girls care more about love and the quality of relationships, in part because of their "specific anatomical–physiological characteristics"'.[4] Fillod's response was to take up the cutting-edge tools of 3D-printing available to her as an engineer, to powerfully bring to light an anatomy that she herself inhabited, but was visibly absent.

Free to download, Fillod's life-size model is a digitised, cutting-edge method for showing and disseminating anatomically correct information, allowing women all over the world to look at their own biology – real, material, life-sized. Undeniable. Incontestable. Like the milk ducts in musculature that, at the start of this book (see page 5), we saw went viral, here we have an expanded example of the role that digital technology can play in consciousness-raising about women's bodies.

Besides the role in teaching all women about their own bodies, with this real-life model of the clitoris in hand, no scientist will be able to ignore the scientific reality of an organ that deserves to be studied in its own right. The idea that the penis is more visible and therefore more sexual is not new – scientists throughout history have dismissed the clitoris as fantastical or deviant or both. The renowned medieval scholar Magnus considered the clitoris as homologous to the penis. In the sixteenth century, the anatomist Vesalius argued that the clitoris did not appear in 'normal' women.[5] The *Malleus Maleficarum*, a 1486 guide for finding witches, suggested the clitoris was the 'devil's treat' and if found on a woman it would prove her status as a witch. In the 1800s, women diagnosed with 'hysteria' were given clitoridectomies (had their clitorises excised).

To see how these scientific artefacts of women's asexuality were exertions of patriarchal power over subjugated populations, you only need to follow the logic to its extreme. A racialised hierarchy was established through nineteenth-century anatomical science, where externalised and more visible labia were associated with the bodies of women of colour and linked to sexual deviance. This placed Black women at the bottom of a stratified system that used biological information to establish the scientific image of the 'normal' vagina in opposition to the abnormality of an excluded and oppressed population.[6] Rendering female genitalia invisible was very much a part of establishing a world order built on the desires of men and not just the denial of women's wants, but also, ingeniously, that women should have desires at all.

In the 1980s, while Dodson was educating women about their bodies, other feminists worked to introduce the clitoral anatomy into science books. In 1981, the Federation of Feminist Women's Health Clinics created anatomically correct images of the clitoris, published in their guide for women, *A New View of a Woman's Body*. Fillod's model builds on this legacy and reveals that the work in educating women about the clitoris and, along with it, their sexuality is not done.

The idea that sex is all about men, not women, remains equally prevalent in the recent history of scientific research on the clitoris. The first comprehensive anatomical study of the clitoris was led by urologist Professor Helen O'Connell and published in 1998.[7] Much later, in a subsequent 2005 study, she examined the clitoris under MRI.[8] These studies showed that it was not just a small nub of erectile tissue, often dubbed 'pea-sized'. Instead, it was an otherworldly shape, with the nerve-rich glands merely the external protrusion of an organ that extended beneath the pubic bone and wrapped around the vaginal opening, with bulbs that become engorged when aroused.

Despite the discovery, in the twenty or so years since O'Connell's ground-breaking study was released, clitoral anatomy remains largely absent from the medical curriculum – and from medical research. A literature review conducted by O'Connell's team for her editorial in the *Australian and New Zealand Journal of Obstetrics and Gynaecology* found just eleven articles on anatomical dissection of the clitoris had been published worldwide since 1947. Eleven. Hundreds more mentioned clitoral anatomy only as it related to procedures to restore sensation following a cliteradectomy, or female genital mutilation.[9] The work that has been done, though, reveals the essential role of the clitoris in female orgasm in the process also debunking the existence of the long-sought-after G-spot.[10]

So when, in 2017, Fillod decided to produce her 3D-model, there was a fascinating, albeit fractured and sporadic scientific literature to draw upon, just waiting for an innovative scientist to put it to new use. The 3D-format utilised by Fillod allowed her to demonstrate boldy the real size and shape of the clitoris, thus blasting through common misconceptions about the supposedly inconspicuous, underdeveloped organ.

The model strikingly shows that a life-size clitoris is about ten centimetres long, from the tip to the glands at the end of one 'crus' (or leg), and that it is shaped like a wishbone. The size and shape present an anatomical reality that is more difficult to ignore than a drawing, definitely an off-the-cuff footnote amid a sea of drawings of penises. As the American Urological Association argued in 2005, 'It is impossible to convey clitoral anatomy in a single diagram.'[11] In the age of 3D-printing technology though, that is no longer a reason to omit the clitoris from sex education or from scientific research.

This is the power of new technology in bringing the dimensions of biology that matter to non-male bodies to light. Here, Fillod, an interdisciplinary researcher, claimed the new technological possibilities available to her and put them to use. She *used* the science available to her and so demonstrated, by representing the clitoris from this informed and multi-skilled perspective, what the scientific depictions were missing. Technology allowed her to test out and demonstrate the findings in the scientific literature. In this technologised age, we have these options and opportunities, when we invite engineers and other skilled professionals into the building of medicine, to construct different stories that challenge the status quo.

Fillod's model has been taken up by sex therapists, sex educators, school nurses, biology teachers and sex-information institutions, all using the model to teach different stories about female sexuality, showing how their experience of sex is as biological and real as the male. And showing also, how much there is yet to discover. Technological invention becomes reinvention when new hands takes it up to do the talking. That is how the clitoris lands, suddenly unrecognisable like an alien spaceship, inviting researchers to explore it anew.

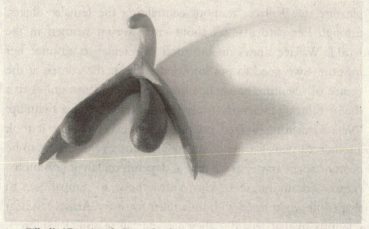

Fillod's 3D-printed clitoris has been used in sex education lessons in French schools from primary level onwards since September 2016.[12]

Fillod's model is not the only reinvented clitoris out there. Images of the clitoris are proliferating, and with them a new alliance of storytellers is forming. Dodson's path from erotic art to anatomical empowerment is recapitulated in the role that art today is playing in raising awareness about the clitoris. The nexus between art and science should by now not be surprising – throughout this book we have seen how ideas shape science and, when it comes to ideas, art is a powerful cultural resource.

CLITERACY – pleasure for everyone

A veritable movement has burgeoned around O'Connell's scientific work bringing the clitoris to light. In 2012, the US-based artist Sophia Wallace created the campaign 'CLITERACY'. Echoing Dodson's philosophy, the project's manifesto read: 'CLITERACY upholds that all bodies are entitled to pleasure, which is fundamental to full citizenship.'[13] Centralising female pleasure, to Wallace, is about centralising the female subject, through her clitoris – it's about empowering women in the world. Wallace draws on the tools of science to advance her mission – we need to put knowledge about the clitoris at the centre of scientific research. Only Wallace too recognises that the usefulness of scientific tools depends on who takes them up: 'Neil Armstrong walked on the moon in 1969, but it took another 29 years for the complete anatomy of the clitoris to be proven.' Space travel, as we noted, depends on adept communicators, communicators who know how to empathise, to shapeshift when faced with unfamiliar territory. Artists can help scientists in that regard – they are after all seasoned explorers, practised in rendering the familiar unfamiliar.

The term 'CLITERACY' captures this move towards collaboration perfectly – when the authoritative literacy of science places the clitoris, symbolic for the female subject, at its core, we have a science that works with women to tell scientific stories that serve them well. Ones that tackle the unknowns about their bodies that they need answered in order to move freely in this world.

The 'literacy' in 'CLITERACY' also points to other important tools – those of reading and writing. We often forget that these are tools we have developed, that we have learnt to use, because we are taught them at such a young age. Yet these are the unknown knowns that guide our understanding of the world, so engrained we forget that they are the lens through which we look. Like gender, once we render this perspective visible, we may start to question just who gets to use them, just who gets to determine *how* they are used. Who has that power.

Different people can become literate, using the tool of literacy to tell different stories – this can be playful, entertaining, fun *and* scientific, because in rendering the familiar unknown, they are speaking to the old voices, asking them to collaborate, to use what they know, to work together on shared unknowns. As with the best sex, in this collaborative activity, scientists and non-scientists make themselves mutually vulnerable, as they explore *together* where their tools take them. Vulnerability makes for good science and good education too – Gwyneth Paltrow's best moments and undoubtedly those that will be most helpful to her audience were when she stopped shouting 'vagina!' at people and made herself vulnerable, when she talked to Dodson and her colleagues about the blocks and pressures she felt when it came to her own sexuality. This is true exploration because it is true exposure to the wonders of the unknown. We need to demand this from scientists and medical professionals too. When it masters the tools of collaborative storytelling, science will go further than it can imagine, because when scientists offer their tools to a new generation of storytellers, when they offer to assist them in answering the questions they ask, it wins not just authority but trust. A communal science of storytelling, a science based on 'CLITERACY', that is the science that will loop twice around the clitoris, past the moon and into a dimension yet unknown.

Yet despite the potential of CLITERACY for astronomical leaps towards medical emancipation, this comes with the same old words of caution. There is of course the potential for this celebration and visibility of female anatomy and a push for a better understanding of its parts to morph into something different. We have to be careful not to replace the kind of systemic change needed in medicine, the healthcare system and society with the so-called 'sexual liberation' of individual women.

Rather than calling for social change, the risk is that this narrative spins into insidious pressure and coercion to abide by a heteronormative version of sexuality according to patriarchal scripts. This has been a critique of second wave feminists championing sex as the path to feminist emancipation – and this should not morph into pressure for women to perform desires they may not feel. It should demand that women are sexually open to be liberated.

It is possible that in adopting the shock tactics of CLITERACY, we transform a space dedicated to male desire into an environment that is equally hostile to expressions of vulnerability. It is the same tendency we have seen in femtech and GripTok to advocate for female health in a loud and overtly sexualised way that isn't necessarily true to female desire. CLITERACY is about fostering a new kind of visibility, not displacing one totalising worldview with another. Like Betty's vibrator, CLITERACY is a tool we can use to generate options for women that will be as useful as the difference it makes to their lives.

With an eye to the future, Alli Sebastian Wolf, a Sydney-based artist, created the Glitoris, an 100–1 scale anatomically correct twinkling gold clitoris, in 2017. The Glitoris can be hung in a gallery but achieved viral fame when Wolf took it to the Women's March, Mardi Gras and other public events, accompanied by the so-called 'Cliterati' – Sebastian Wolf and friends in gold unitards and blue wigs.

'A lot of people just thought it was a golden-y squid creature, a lot of people thought it was lungs, or a dragonfly, or testicles,' Wolf said.[14] 'I met a couple of OB-GYNs who hadn't known about it until the sculpture, which is horrifying.'

The hope, for Wolf, is that her art will destigmatise discussions about the clitoris among scientists and non-scientists alike – the outlandishness of her model paradoxically normalises discussions about the clitoris. 'It will hopefully get to the point where my art is totally irrelevant,' she says. Like gender, like the other consciousness-raising concepts and images we've seen – all navigational tools on the path to a more inclusive science – the Glitoris, too, is 'designed to be deleted'.

Wallace made a similar point when interviewed about her own art. When asked why she chose the name CLITERACY for her movement, she replied: 'It's that once somebody is taught to read, they can't be untaught. Once you're literate, that's the end of it. There's no going back. And that's what I wanted for CLITERACY – you don't have to like it, you don't have to like the art or the message or the messenger – but once you have the facts and the information, you can't give them back. You don't have to do anything with the knowledge, but you can't give it back.'[15] CLITERACY can't be unlearnt.

Perhaps this is the most futuristic prospect we have come across on our journey through medicine. Besides 3D-printed clitorises, besides the reinvented vibrators, virtual reality sex environments designed by women,[16] sex robots (pretty unconvincing substitutes for humans to date) and other digitised gadgets that go beyond vaginal stimulation but work with the body in other ways, challenging heteronormative models of sex,[17] that may help women explore their bodies today, perhaps of all of them the most mind-blowing intervention will be universal CLITERACY. Once CLITERACY has been fully integrated into our curricula, it will be naturalised, a tool that seems innate, that shapes everything we say and see and think. CLITERACY by this point will be a redundant concept, synonymous with literacy itself. And so, stories become reality.

This new literacy isn't just about the clitoris: CLITERACY represents a whole new science in which non-male biology is woven into scientific knowledge. This highly advanced science will incorporate different storytellers, working together to tell 'clitoral' tales that transport us to a shared unknown – outlandish worlds where science has the most to offer, where it shows us something new.

With Cliteracy integrated into its DNA, into its hormones, into its muscles and bones and all its biological systems, science will be defined by a new unknown known – that good science is feminist through and through.

Chapter 13

Biotech

[W]e are all chimeras, theorised and fabricated hybrids of machine and organism; in short, we are cyborgs.

Donna Haraway[1]

To me, stories are where scientific possibilities are born, and the more creatively we can imagine our world through fiction, the farther we'll go. Donna Haraway is one of my favourite cultural critics of science and technology. She embraces the potential that the genre of science fiction has to reimagine society. She envisions possibility.

Throughout this last section, the potential of new technology lies not just in its practical applications but in its power to disrupt the stories about gender roles that we have come to accept – about the role of reproduction in a woman's life and her role in society. Science fictions – whether written or suggested by the possible uses of a new technology – have always given me hope that my body may be more accepted, may be valued differently and receive better care, not just superficially by including women in existing research or clinical trials, but much more permanently, by drawing us all into new imaginative landscapes, a future of scientific potential that does away with the limitations of the gender roles we are assigned. Haraway's work exemplifies that potential. So much so, that in 1985, she introduced her own piece of science fiction into the usually matter of fact and formulaic journal articles of the social science canon with a piece published in the *Socialist Review*.

The title?

'A Cyborg Manifesto.'

Haraway used this piece of writing to develop the metaphor of the cyborg. Not just as a futuristic robot found in science fiction films, but, among other things, as real, living people whose physical abilities have been extended beyond their normal human limitations by mechanical elements built into their bodies. Today, people sporting bionic limbs and artificial pacemakers, for example, give us many creative renditions of cyborgs.

The term 'cyborg' was originally coined in the context of space travel, in a 1960 paper by the scientists Manfred Clynes and Nathan Kline,[2] who imagined that through a combination of technology, drugs and space, humans would surmount their natural and material conditions to ameliorate the symptoms of everyday reality – and in doing so, create a better one. The 1960s were a time when scientists in computer technology were expanding and exploring the applications of the wired-up feedback loops of their cybernetic systems; they conceived of merging the two into one – a cybernetic organism. A new frontier in science. At the time, cyborgs were second only to space travel in terms of the horizons they offered to scientists and science fiction enthusiasts alike. In fact, the exploration of the relationships between inner and outer space, mind and matter, body and technology went hand in hand.

Haraway drew on this world-building potential of the image

of a technologised person to challenge some of the most rigid definitions, based on oppositions that defined the world as people knew it. In doing so, she asked humanity to seriously consider how it could reimagine a world based on affinities across these boundaries, and with it, a different way of doing science, of exploring the unknown.

While a cyborg might seem a far cry from 'natural' humanity, Haraway argued that the boundaries between technology and people are not so clear-cut as we might first believe. In the modern world, we are always connected to technology, some basic, some advanced, and we are all integrated in complex networks of connections between humans and technology that make us who we are. For Haraway, the realities of contemporary life simply included a relationship between people and technology so intimate that it would no longer be possible to tell where we ended and machines began.

We might like to think that we humans can be 'natural', that technology is 'other' to us, but we exist in a system that is anything but natural, and when we start to consider our medicine in this way, we'll come to see our own bodies as cyborg systems, too; as connected to medical technologies that are often imperceptible but shape who we are. We are fed on the products of agribusiness, kept healthy – or damaged – by pharmaceuticals and altered by medical procedures.

When people describe something as natural, they're saying that it's just how the world is, that we can't change it. Women for generations were told that they were 'naturally' weak, submissive, overemotional and incapable of abstract thought. That it was 'in our nature' to be mothers rather than corporate raiders, to prefer parlour games to particle physics. If all these things are natural, they're unchangeable. End of story. If, however, women (and men) aren't natural but are constructed, like a cyborg, then, given the right tools, we can all be *recon*structed – conceptually and physically. Our ideas about gender roles supposedly engrained in our 'natural' biology can be reassessed.

Just as in the Bones chapter, earlier in the book, we saw how social beliefs lead to biological tendencies that come to be seen as inherent to biology, changing our social beliefs about gender can lead us to develop new interventions that physically change biology. Basic assumptions suddenly come into question, such as whether it's natural to have a society based on violence and the domination of one group by another. Maybe humans are biologically destined to fight wars and trash the environment. Maybe we're not.

Feminists around the world have seized on this possibility. Cyberfeminism – not a term Haraway uses, but coined later, in the early 1990s – is based on the idea that, in conjunction with technology, it's possible to construct your identity, your sexuality, even your gender, just as you please. This is why Haraway likes science fiction. It's why I like science fiction. The slippage between realities invites us to be both interested in and critical towards the worlds we inhabit, to entertain what we have rendered inconceivable and to interrogate alternative realities as possibilities – as versions of a sci-fi story that could be told differently and, in turn, full of other social possibilities.

In the same way that science is a tool we can use to build better worlds, fictions can be used to imagine the scientific possibilities that need to be imagined first, in order for scientists to bring them into being. Neither is inherently progressive and both rely on people putting them to use in the best interest of the members of society they prioritise. These science fictions are social fictions about imagining, about creating better worlds. About possibilities.

Weird science is good science

I'd like to paint a picture for you of an image, equally cyborg and sci-fi, a strange uninhabited planet, hollow inside. Beneath its surface, a fluffy, living lining is shed each month, only then magically regenerates with not the trace of a scar across its surface. It's a mesmerising landscape, re-emerging, spiralling blood vessels sprawled like the work of a delicate seamstress across its surface. This is the womb. And it looks very different the more you learn about it. Its mystery doesn't reflect a specif-ically female mystique, only the infinitely receding horizons of every part of the human body, which always leaves more for scientists to unearth, and of which they will only see what they understand – and understand what they first imagine they might want to see.

The womb looks even less recognisable in the lab-grown microcosms of Dr Linda Griffith's lab in The MIT Center for Gynaepathology Research. Dr Griffith is a bioengineer by training, sculpting organs using basic biological building blocks. In 1997, she helped create an iconic creature, the earmouse, by injecting a human ear-shaped scaffold with carti-lage from a cow's knee and growing it on the back of a lab mouse.[3] With this early cyborg of an animal and human-like structures merging to challenge our definitions of the bounda-ries between natural and technologically assisted body parts and between animal and human, Dr Griffith was already on the path to *showing* us, demonstrating biologically why our known biological categories, when opened up to true cutting-edge scientific investigation, do not hold.

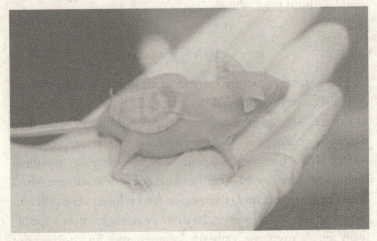

Mouse with engineered ear on the back,
otherwise known as 'earmouse'.

Though the earmouse might seem a far cry from the sort of medicine we might want to consider practically, Dr Griffith has brought her background in bioengineering to the challenge of understanding endometriosis, that incredibly widespread chronic disorder in which tissue similar to that which normally lines the uterus instead grows outside it.

Endometriosis, it is thought, affects over 10% of all women, and has been discussed throughout this book – and, indeed, throughout the media – as an emblem for the women-specific diseases that have been trivialised and ignored in male-centric medicine. In 2021, Dr Griffith and colleagues published a paper reporting how they had created bits of bioengineered tissue that would allow researchers to visualise the growth of lesions in three dimensions, revealing processes of gland and nerve formation that happen inside the uterus, allowing them to determine the role of immune cells, inflammation and hormones in the disease.[4] Like the Smart Tampon, the endometriosis model was lauded in part for its diagnostic potential for a neglected 'female' disease. But beyond that, it was particularly exciting because it showed that the endometrium was relevant to other disciplines not traditionally associated with women's health, such as immune function or tissue regeneration. Dr Griffith's work, as we'll see, moves the symbolic heart of woman as a reproductive vessel into other areas of science, expanding the landscape of women's health beyond reproduction, and also connecting other fields of medicine to the study of reproduction, morphing them into more than their male-centric shadows.

Dr Griffith's background in constructing boundary-breaking biological creatures has shaped her breakthroughs in the science of endometriosis in more ways than one. Crucially, it has led her to irrevocably shatter the narrow definition of the uterus as a reproductive organ and so, perhaps, of the woman as a reproductive vessel too. First of all, her expertise in constructing biological models has allowed her to grow uterine organoids – tiny domed droplets, with glands that look like swirling craters – from the uterine cells of endometriosis patients. These 'patient avatars' are ideal tools for testing potential new treatments for the disease: biologically, they are closer to human uterine cells than those of mice (which don't naturally menstruate). And they enable researchers to sidestep the ethical issues that would arise with human trials.

Just like stem cells since HeLa have given scientists new possibilities for understanding the behaviour of cells without having to test directly on human embryos or tissue, these (dare

I say) cyborg creatures allow scientists across disciplines to unite over shared models to tackle the questions that matter to women, but also allow them to imagine a way of avoiding the demands that the extraction of biological materials for science continue to put on women and their bodies. The models have allowed Dr Griffith to compare them with real patients in order to start to explain the biological mechanisms underlying the dynamism of the endometrium's regeneration, understanding when and how it goes wrong and why.

Her work signals the possibility of an end to an era that saw menstruation as a period of waste and decay deemed uninteresting by a science obsessed with the woman as a baby-maker. The uterus does much more than bear children it turns out. It is inherently regenerative, is shed and recovered almost every month (when no fertilised egg implants) and so it offers a window onto biological systems other than reproduction, such as tissue generation, scarless wound healing and immune function. These biological entities, as lab-made reconstructions of a human organ, are themselves already cyborgs that, like the earmouse, challenge the boundaries between humans and technology. And this time, the cyborg is an inherently feminist tool, with the potential to upturn past gender categories, to render the biologically natural unfamiliar and to ask what new functions we can unearth in what now appears as unexplored territory.

The biotech endometrium will go on to lead scientists far beyond the narrow category of reproduction and, in doing so, will form different associations between the womb and woman and her role in society. One area where the endometrium has much to offer is in stem cell science. Prolific in the uterine lining, stem cells might help explain why with endometriosis, lesions appear throughout the body, in the lungs, eyes, spine and brain, as it is possible that stem cells from the uterus circulate the body. Uterine stem cells can also be harnessed in regenerative medicine. They are, as we have already seen, readily accessible. Recent research has shown that they can be grown into new neurons and insulin-making cells to treat diseases like Parkinson's and diabetes.

In research conducted in a reproductive sciences laboratory at Yale, scientists unexpectedly discovered on extracting stem cells from human endometrial tissue that these cells could differentiate into dopaminergic neurons: the brain cells that are lost in Parkinson's disease leading symptoms like tremor, speech difficulty and poor balance that characterise the disease. These scientists, working on the endometrium, were surprised to find that their research could inform treatment for a neurogenerative condition far outside of the usual purview of reproductive science. The team went on to show that these neurons can boost the fallen dopamine levels in mice and primates with mild Parkinson's disease and to investigate how other symptoms of the disease might be alleviated by introducing these cells.[5] Taylor and his team also found that they could coax the uterine stem cells into producing insulin. They introduced these differentiated versions of the stem cells into diabetic mice where they kept producing insulin, stabilising their blood glucose, providing potential treatment for the disease in humans.[6]

The stem cells' tendency to differentiate into dopaminergic neurons is as yet unexplained, but Taylor and his colleagues have also coaxed the cells into becoming insulin-producing beta cells. Trials in mouse models have used endometrial stem cells to produce beta cells that continued producing insulin and stabilised blood-glucose levels within five weeks when injected into diabetic mice.

Like the Smart Tampon, the bioengineered endometrium is a repurposing of a long-standing sign of womanhood in the form of a biological demonstration of the ways in which this organ has different functions and can be understood in different contexts. Further work Dr Griffith has done investigates how the uterus interacts with other organs throughout the body. Her background is in systems engineering and central to this discipline is the understanding that all the systems of the body interact. You cannot merely take out one part and expect it to function or make sense in isolation; that mistake is at the root of male-centric medicine to begin with; the assumption that the only difference between men and women was down to their reproductive systems, and so that the female reproductive system can be studied in isolation. But as we now know, the body is defined by a set of interacting, interconnected systems. To capture this idea, Dr Griffith and her team connect their models to other organs like bone marrow, gut and liver – and also hope to seed them with blood vessels, nerve cells and immune cells. In this way of doing science, researchers learn more about their object of study by complicating the picture, rather than simplifying it. They start asking how the world they thought they understood connects to other worlds.

In 1999 a picture of the earmouse accompanied a full-page ad in the *New York Times* signed by a list of groups including the Foundation on Economic Trends, the Institute for Agriculture and Trade Policy and Mothers for Natural Law, among others. The ad was titled 'Who Plays God in the 21st Century?'. Bioengineered creations have repeatedly evoked this question to the point of cliché. *Brave New World* is the literary comparison of choice here – a dystopia, written in 1931, in which author Aldous Huxley predicted a society where humans are genetically engineered for commercial and industrial purposes. People don't protest because they are designed 'to love their servitude'. 'Has that already happened to us? Not yet! Call us,' the writers of the article reassure the readers, in their effort to campaign for 'safety requirements for biotechnology'.[7]

The authors misconstrue the earmouse as a product of genetic engineering, among other inaccuracies such as the idea that biotech companies are 'blithely removing components of human beings, and other creatures, and treating us all like auto parts at a swap meet'. The ears on the mice, as we know, weren't taken from human bodies, and were, instead, grown by the host's body itself. Yet the subtext of the piece is clear: panic in the face of scientific advancements we, as a society, have not learnt to manage, scientific power that could be exploited in the wrong hands. Responses like these overlook in their conflation of science fiction futures and exploitation that science – and people – have already been exploited for the benefit of select groups of society. We've already seen the multitude of ways in which diverse groups in society have suffered and continue to suffer as the result of a male bias in science and medicine.

But scholars like Donna Haraway, and many feminist writers of science fiction, show that the advance of science in imaginatively challenging directions provides an opportunity to reflect on the moral, social, political and economic choices driving this science. The striking appearance of an earmouse, a lab-grown human or the palpable trade in physical body parts and tissues command us to answer a question that has previously remained implicit yet opaque at the heart of science: who benefits from scientific advancement? Whose bodies and tissues are we using and how do we value them? Whose diseases are we preventing or curing? And why?

In January of 2018, doctors in China and Japan published a study of children with one malformed ear and one healthy ear. Over the course of the study, they scanned the healthy ears and used mirrored versions of those scans to recreate and produce 3D-biodegradable printed scaffolds to which they added cartilage cells from their patients.[8] In this way, they were able to give the children new ears. This is the most direct clinical outcome that can be easily connected to the work done on the earmouse, but the endometriosis model is another, as are the insights in regenerative medicine, immune and stem cell science that have resulted, and will result in years to come.

The directions science takes are unpredictable, the connections and interactions of cyborg systems always are, but, like human bodies, they are guided by principles. Choice, once again, emerges as the most important principle of human growth. The choices of the scientists in the questions they choose to explore, the choices of governments and policymakers as they fund and prioritise research, and all of them as they choose who to give choice to. The power of cyborg biology is not about brave new worlds but about better worlds, worlds in which society takes responsibility for the direction science takes. A world in which high-tech uteruses prompt regeneration.

Chapter 14

Artificial Wombs

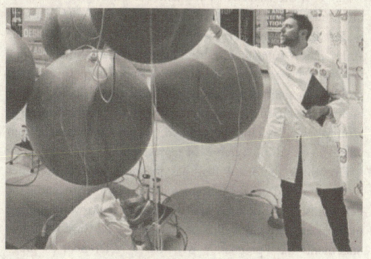

The prototype artificial womb as displayed at
the Reprodutopia exhibition at Droog gallery in
Amsterdam. Photograph by Nichon Glerum.[1]

A mother who undergoes a nine-month pregnancy is likely to feel
that the product of all that pain and discomfort 'belongs' to her.
— Shulamith Firestone[2]

In the age of engineered biology, artists, feminists, authors and
scientists alike have not only imagined how the womb could

be repurposed and studied in fields other than reproductive biology, breaking with the limiting associations between female biology and child-carrier, they have also asked how we can take the womb as a childbearing vessel and extract it from the female body. They have thus challenged the naturalisation of women as biological baby-makers by making gestation everybody's business. Behold, another otherworldly planet floating in unfamiliar space. The artificial womb.

In 1970, the Canadian-born feminist and writer Shulamith Firestone painted a radical picture of the future of women's bodies. In her feminist manifesto, *The Dialectic of Sex: The Case for Feminist Revolution*, Firestone suggested that women's childbearing role was at the core of female oppression. To solve the problem of gender inequality, she said, they had to replace biological reproduction with ectogenesis, that is gestation in an artificial womb. This, she argued, would free women from what she called the 'tyranny of reproduction'.

Firestone's rhetorical flair has in some ways tainted her legacy and led to a misinterpretation of the meaning of her words. The book sparked widespread controversy among mainstream critics as well as her fellow second wave feminists. Statements like 'pregnancy is barbaric', references to pregnancy as the 'temporary deformation of the body of the individual for the sake of the species' and descriptions of giving birth as being 'like shitting a pumpkin' undoubtedly alienated women for whom pregnancy had been a rewarding or important part of their lives.

Firestone's claims, however, centred around the idea that reproductive technologies that included the artificial womb held the potential to increase women's reproductive choices and autonomy. Firestone pointed to a time before effective contraception was widely available, when women would often become trapped in an ongoing cycle of pregnancy, childbirth and nursing their children. This, she argued, meant that women became dependent on men for sustenance and shelter and were excluded from other social functions. It created a class division that preceded those between rich and poor: namely, that between male producers and female reproducers. Reliable contraception, safe abortion and emerging IVF technologies offered the potential for women to control their own wombs. These could liberate women from both medicine and politics controlled by men which, for example, only allowed contraception to married women. The artificial womb was an *in-extremis* expression of a reality, a kind of rhetorical device that allowed Firestone to picture a world in which women were freed from their forced and tightly controlled labour as reproducers. If childbearing was no longer the domain of women but a collective responsibility, women would be free to take on other roles in society and could develop their identities beyond the walking wombs that the present social structure made them out to be.

The artificial womb, with its promises of gestating a foetus outside of the female body, *conceptually* severed the reproductive capacity from natural female biology. It is an idea we can use to imagine a world in which female bodies are not defined by their role in reproduction. In medicine, too, the artificial womb can be used as a tool, a useful starting point for rethinking the needs of female bodies when these are no longer conflated with a natural, inevitable and sacrificial form of childbearing that deprioritises the health and wellbeing of the mother. For me, the interesting point Firestone raises is how technologised childbirth moves childbirth into the public sphere as an important and valuable activity. If we imagine gestation happening in centralised locations rather than 'hidden' inside homes, reproduction explicitly becomes the point of national importance it always should have been, and so perhaps we will start to adequately value it, fund it, research it, support it and regulate it.

Womb 2.0

The artificial wombs being developed right now will not replace childbearing in the way that Firestone envisioned. Researchers currently working on prototypes in the United States, Australia and Japan envision that the artificial womb could eventually be used to support babies who are born prematurely with continued gestation, rather than in neonatal intensive care where there is still a high risk of mortality and serious morbidity.

In reality, then, these wombs will be used much along the same lines as the endometriosis models in the previous chapters – they'll be repurposed, here more narrowly, within the domain of childbirth, but nonetheless will come to represent a distinct stage in the process outside the mother's womb – a womb 2.0. This is where we come full circle, we return to the ways in which taking reproduction seriously will move us through and beyond this sphere as the defining aspect of the female body in medicine and society by making reproduction a societal not a women's issue.

The human-made womb will demonstrate the ways in which reproduction is cyborg; that is, it relies on technology and assistance that isn't just biological but rooted in social systems. In this less direct way, even this less radical implementation of the artificial womb begins to demonstrate the possibility raised by Firestone – that when reproduction is moved, even in part, out of the female body and into communally owned incubators, we command the world to see itself through a reproductive lens – a lens that will eventually be as natural as the male default. Reproduction will become an important dimension of any social or medical question, just as money and labour are now. The cyborg womb demonstrates the same potential that has animated me in writing this book – that when we take gendered ideas seriously, by which I mean, when we choose to investigate them rather than take them as a given, we bring them into mainstream medicine as the new status quo, where we can be guided by an understanding that 'women's issues' are everyone's issue.

The research into the possibility of using artificial wombs to support premature babies is well under way. In 2019, the Australian and Japanese scientists repeated the success of keeping extremely premature lambs alive inside an artificial womb environment until they were ready to survive on their own. Those researchers are now developing a treatment strategy for premature babies between twenty and twenty-three weeks of gestation. The prototype being developed by Dutch researchers is especially interesting, going so far as to replicate the sound of a mother's heartbeat inside the 'biobag'. In this EU-funded $3 million project at the Eindhoven University of Technology, the team aims to develop an artificial womb for preterm babies between twenty-four and twenty-eight weeks of gestation by 2024.

Their design encompasses a fluid-based environment that mimics that of the natural womb, where the baby receives oxygen and nutrients through an artificial placenta that is connected to the baby's umbilical cord. The team wants to design a 'perfectly natural' artificial womb. The team uses 3D-printing technology to produce both the wombs and the artificial babies to test in them. These 'mannequins' are equipped with sensors that can replicate the environment a foetus experiences inside the mother's womb – including the soothing sound of her heartbeat.

The emphasis by the Dutch team on replicating the kind of intimacy that, they assume, exists between mother and foetus in pregnancy points to the tensions at the heart of designing these new technologies. Even in this limited application of supporting preterm babies, the simulation of a heartbeat in the artificial environment points to a palpable, and somewhat eerie, absence: the mother's body. What assumptions about pregnancy are being encoded in the designs of artificial wombs? Who decides what aspects of pregnancy are important, what ideas about female biology we retain, the role of female bodies in the process? While technologically separated, ideas about the role of a mother still seem to be at the conceptual heart of scientists' thinking about the artificial womb.

Some have questioned these assumptions about 'normal' gestation, in particular the emphasis sceptics have placed on the ways in which the technology might disrupt the mother–child bond. Professor of Philosophy Anna Smajdor, for example, has provocatively challenged this emphasis on a biologically rooted connection between mother and child during gestation.[3] She makes the point that those who argue for the primacy of the gestational bond do a disservice to all the step- and adoptive parents who love their children dearly, as well as the fathers who love their children as much as mothers do. She also argues that conversely, the physical connection of mothers with their babies does not guarantee a loving bond. Many women don't bond with their naturally born children (it is no surprise that this in itself is a taboo subject in a society that shames women who do fall into the limiting definitions of motherhood it holds). Smajdor even argues that the processes of giving birth we take as natural are partly to blame. Postpartum depression, for example, affects 13% (undoubtedly a conservative figure given the number of women who will not seek help) of women who give birth and may cause the mother to reject her child or refuse to nurture them, and that would not be a risk factors if babies were artificially gestated.

It is also worth acknowledging here that the artificial womb is just the next step in an ongoing technologisation of reproduction, in many cases already assisted through scientific intervention. In traditional pregnancies as well as pregnancies by in vitro fertilisation or surrogacy, many of the most important bonding moments occur when parents see their growing embryo or foetus on a screen. The first ultrasound or the image of an embryo being selected for IVF are becoming culturally significant moments in all forms of pregnancy, which depend little on whether their child exists inside a parent's own body or not. Smajdor concludes that there are many permutations of childrearing in our society, and that it is dubious to locate some kind of mystic essence of parenthood in gestation and childbirth when they cannot be directly associated with the development of the living bond or even benefits to the child.

While there are challenges to developing artificial wombs that replicate the physiological environment needed to sustain a growing foetus, including, for example, the correct supply of nutrients, submersion in sterile and warm fluid and the connection to an umbilical system, we need to think carefully about the emphasis we place on a woman carrying a child inside her own body, and to what extent this preoccupation derives from a social and increasingly outdated idea about the gendered roles women should play as mothers in society.

While it is hard to deny the benefits of supporting the fifteen million babies who are born prematurely each year and are likely to experience serious respiratory, cardiovascular, visual and hearing problems and learning disabilities, we might evoke Firestone's troubled ghost here to ask what assumptions are being designed into these replicas of the female body. Will we see in them just a recapitulation of male power over women's childbearing choices? Or will they be liberating, offering women agency through more reproductive choice?

As the Dutch team's design choices already suggest, the answer to that question, as has been the case throughout this book, depends very much on the ideas we cultivate through the science of artificial wombs, as much as the technological possibilities themselves. Firestone herself warned that artificial wombs had the ability to repress as much as liberate, depending on who had control of the science.

For this reason, it is notable – and problematic to me – that the team working on the Dutch prototype are all male. As we have seen, the overrepresentation of male scientists in medicine shapes the priorities and questions that dominate the field. It has, for example, already been noted in popular media that the flesh-coloured balls of the Dutch prototype resemble dangling testicles more than they do the shape of a womb. Likenesses have been drawn to the 'alchemical homunculus', an image developed by medieval alchemists as they tried to conjure up miniature versions of themselves in glass bottles. The tiny men, they believed, might even be spiritually superior versions of a person. Some feminists, you might imagine, see the artificial womb as a continuation of this history of men seizing control over reproduction, rendering women's role obsolete, at the same time as they create idealised versions of the human in a distinctly male form. I can't say that they are wrong, only point to the possibilities and the necessary discussions that will determine the role we imagine and create for the artificial womb in our society today.

Whether one sees testicles or not, it is clear that there is work to be done to ensure that artificial wombs don't become, as the rest of medicine arguably has been, a male fantasy. If artificial womb technology is adequately developed, it may, in the future, offer new options and choices for the owners of female bodies to bear children in new ways. It may even offer options in fertility treatment, for people unable to gestate naturally, including infertile women and couples, but also single people and members of the LGBTQIA+ community, creating an alternative to surrogacy, with its legal complications, or uterus transplantation, with its medical risks.

In the end, the emancipatory potential of the technology will depend on how the ideas mould how it is used. If, for example, the option to gestate in an artificial womb does eventually come to be a viable alternative to natural gestation, will the women who choose to do it the old-fashioned way still receive the support they require? Will medical research prioritise women's health in pregnancy when it has the option to study foetal development in an environment completely severed from the mother's body?

As well as the threat of further neglect of female medical needs, there is the possibility that the artificial womb will lead to greater control in how pregnancies and pregnant people are treated. The option of an alternative, perhaps even safer version of pregnancy might lead to the argument that pregnant people should be more closely monitored, again undermining biological mothers' rights to make decisions regarding their own pregnancies. Claire Horn, Doctor of Law at Birkbeck, University of London, has shown that the earliest attempts to create artificial wombs in the 1870s represented an effort to erase the mother from pregnancy, with supposed concerns among many obstetricians 'that mothers themselves, with their unsanitary practices, irresponsible behaviour and anxious fussing, might pose a danger to their infants – a danger that could be curbed by placing the uterus-incubator firmly in the doctors' hands'. We need to be wary of perpetuating these views of women as incapable and their biology as controllable in the design and implementation of the artificial womb today. We need to be attuned to the needs of the owners of bodies who will continue to be neglected or disenfranchised if we maintain these deeply engrained ideas about male control over female reproduction – artificial womb and natural womb alike.

There are also important questions about who would have access to this inevitably expensive reproductive option. Surrogacy researcher and author Sophie Lewis writes in *Full Surrogacy Now*[4] that many thousands of women continue to die due to pregnancy-related complications every year due to social, not simply 'natural', reasons. Gestating can be deadly – largely for political and economic reasons. Typically, safer gestation has always been the privilege of the white and wealthy. There is the real possibility that ectogenesis will further entrench existing inequality in reproduction between those who can afford technological assistance and those who cannot. When it comes to the development of the artificial womb, it's important to know not only who will design and control these technologies but also who will have access; which women will use these technologies under what circumstances.

Medical reports have already shown racial and ethnic disparities in infertility treatments and access to assisted reproductive technologies. In England, a single cycle of IVF treatment can cost up to £5,000, and couples usually require multiple cycles.[5] There is no reason to believe that artificial wombs would be any different. In the worst case, we might imagine a *Handmaid's Tale* scenario, where that inequity in access to healthcare might mean that women who can afford an artificial womb will be able to live their lives unperturbed, while those who cannot might be closely monitored and severely judged in their lifestyle choices to ensure that they are providing optimal conditions for their foetus, given their 'substandard' route to childbearing.

An alternative vision

There is another possible future, however, perhaps less utopian than Firestone's, but one that would be promising for female health. Leaving the radical restructuring of society aside for now, imagine that artificial wombs are introduced into clinical care only as a life-saving alternative to intensive neonatal care. In this case, the severely premature babies born before the crucial twenty-eight-week mark, who usually die, now survive. The further fifteen million (and rising) babies born prematurely worldwide every year will be moved to a new uterine environment where they receive the support they need to develop healthily. Imagine, too, that the scientists and designers involved in developing the prototypes, and the subjects these are then tested on and with, are a broadly representative group of diverse women, shaping the artificial womb and the procedures around it in a way that is beneficial to the needs to female bodies; asking the questions and designing studies that ensure the artificial womb is optimised for mother, child and female bodies everywhere, as their findings reveal new areas of female body-specific research.

Imagine, then, that once the artificial womb is tried and tested and ready for clinical use, the health services or insurers in respective countries decide to provide this new form of neonatal care for free at the point of use. This way, it won't only be the well-to-do with access to this life-saving possibility, but also the low-income and ethnic and racial minority women who make up the majority of mothers who have premature babies, who are often forced to compromise on healthcare, who can give their children a better start to life. The mothers of these premature babies, again, most often those with reduced access to effective healthcare, will also avoid the possible long-term deleterious physical and mental consequences of these preterm births. Perhaps we would live in a world where more of these children would go on to live fulfilling lives with healthy parents, and perhaps their children would go on to do the same.

At present, the development of artificial wombs remains unregulated. While human prototypes have been geared towards supporting preterm babies as described, other groups of scientists are exploring the possibility of full ectogenesis in animals. A handful of reports has recently been published that suggest the potential to transform artificial wombs from laboratory tools for scientists studying early development to a clinical tool used to grow and maintain human embryos from fertilisation until birth. Two of these papers reported the generation of human blastocysts (a mammalian embryo in the first stage of development, when the fertilised egg has grown into a hollow ball, made up of a few hundred cells), not through fertilisation – not even by using the cells of embryos – but by culturing non-embryonic cells under specific conditions to transform them into blastocyst-like structures, called 'blastoids'. In one study, scientists used stem cells derived from an established stem cell line to create the blastoids.[6] In the second study, scientists used adult skin cells and reprogrammed them into blastoids.[7] The third of these articles published in the same issue[8] reported that scientists had developed an artificial womb that sustained the development of early mouse embryos into a foetus that contained fully formed organs. These developments adhere to current legislative restrictions for working on embryos in the lab, but there will need to be discussions on whether the science is ready to support full ectogenesis safely, and whether this is something that we as a society want. The question that is most useful to ask in this case will be the one that underlies much of the science fiction images and feminist writing on the possibilities of artificial wombs, but that is often misconstrued as a question of simply right or wrong.

To me, the legacy of feminist thinking on these matters raises a more important question, rife with possibility, namely: for what purpose? Supporting mothers and premature babies across society is a cause I could get behind; full ectogenesis could offer options to women but will only deliver if the technology is safe and it will also be essential that childbearing is valued. If the technology is taken up not just, as Firestone imagined, to liberate women from childbirth but also to make it a societally valued contribution, then perhaps the appropriate social infrastructure will follow. Women who choose to bear children will be supported – and those who don't will have access to the best of well-funded, cutting-edge science. Perhaps we'll see a society where women aren't defined by their reproductive capacity but are instead supported in it.

The artificial womb can be the symbolic heart of a new body of medicine that incorporates the issues that matter *throughout* its disciplines, that dares to take a different perspective on the medical issues it thought it knew, by incorporating new lenses, new perspectives that matter to female, minority and differently gendered bodies, adding new layers of meaning in the palimpsest of the medical textbook it will never finish writing. The advanced technological possibilities emerging in biotech can help provide these disorientating framings, to urge scientists to venture further. The difference between utopia and dystopia hinges on the social infrastructure we develop alongside the science, and this depends on what we value, who we value, and on how far we allow our minds to wander as we imagine the choices we have, and the choices we want to offer.

Conclusion

It matters what matters we use to think other matters with; it matters what stories we tell to tell other stories with; it matters what knots knot knots, what thoughts think thoughts, what descriptions describe descriptions, what ties tie ties. It matters what stories make worlds, what worlds make stories.

– Donna Haraway[1]

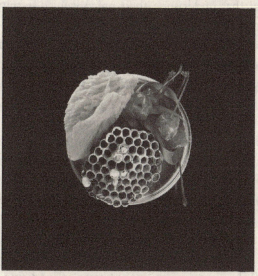

Vanitas (in a Petri dish) 03 by visual artist and Bio Art pioneer, Suzanne Anker.[2]

We all have biology in common. We all inhabit unique biological worlds but we can all relate to what it means to live in and through a body. Science and medicine should have tended to that universal need, but somehow, it has evolved around division instead. At the root of that splintering is a problem of storytelling. Science has been telling stories that falsely claim universal status, while omitting the stories that challenge its power of definition. It's time for that to change.

We see as far as the eye can reach, but the task of science is to imagine where we might reach, given the right tools. That's a highly challenging, deeply creative endeavour, but in this book, I hope to have shown how stories can help. To move beyond their fields' gendered limitations, scientists need to face the outdated stories they have been telling, to start listening to the stories that undermine their preconceived narratives, and to dare to start telling stories too.

The stories in this book about women and about the meaning of their bodies – the stories told in science and art and on the internet – whether pejorative or outlandish, limiting or new, are all hopeful to me.

Stories express the malleable potential of science to evolve as our ideas change. How a model of an endometrium framed as a story about immune function, not just reproduction, has the potential to set scientists on a whole different course, with benefits for everyone's health. We can also read the old stories scientists have told about men and women's bodies, about their sperm and egg cells and the roles they play and reinterpret them to identify the open questions for scientists to explore. This book has been critical of the state of medicine, but it is written from a place of love – a love of the good science can do and a love of the stories we can use to change it by opening up different biological worlds.

The eighteenth-century poet-philosopher Novalis wrote a story about unrequited love or the loss of a loved one symbolised by a blue flower. The 'Blue flower' (*Blaue Blume*) became a central symbol of inspiration in Romanticism. Novalis introduced the symbol into the movement through his unfinished coming-of-age story 'Heinrich von Ofterdingen', in which the young Heinrich dreams about a blue flower following a meeting with a stranger, which calls to him and absorbs his attention. The flower came to stand for desire, love and the metaphysical striving for the infinite and unreachable throughout the movement.

Scientists haven't been able to emulate the blue flower. They've tried many times and many companies have come close, maybe creating a lavender or dark purple one. But the blue flower continues to represent the unattainable – and maybe that's just as well. The very fact that scientists hundreds of years later are drawing on a story, conjured up through a story, to create a horticultural specimen is testament to the sustaining power of stories. The power of the blue flower is no less potent for being imaginary, actually more so, as it sustains scientific inquiry through the ages, reminding us all to continue to interrogate the boundaries of what we know.

The blue flower appears as a symbol in many cultural compositions, as far reaching as Stanley Kubrick's film *Eyes Wide Shut*. Walter Benjamin, influential philosopher, cultural critic and essayist, used it too, interestingly in 'The Work of Art in the Age of Mechanical Reproduction' (1935), where he proposes a theory of art for the age of mass production, an age in which, he argued, a work of art could only be read in context: 'The equipment-free aspect of reality has here become the height of artifice, and the vision of immediate reality the Blue Flower in the land of technology.' In his era, Benjamin argued, art had to be understood in a political context due to the way it was embedded in a highly organised technological system of mass production; artistic expression had lost its sense of immediacy, was no longer pure expression and reality was mediated through these (should I dare mix my critics?) cyborg networks. The blue flower in Benjamin's essay brings us back to the importance of storytelling in science.

Stories show us the world in which science exists, the environment that it inseparable from – the social networks that shape it, the people it serves and excludes, the living, breathing context that makes it. Storytelling and science are drawn together by common images, reflecting the time in their own unique vocabularies, often revealing similar truths – such as the impossibility, given our embeddedness in technological systems, to determine the truth definitively. That the truth in science, as in art, is always framed by a particular perspective, always leaves more to be explained, always remains a blue flower.

This represents the ever-receding horizon of science, its ever-existing potential, but also its ever-limited scope. The antidote – innovations in storytelling. Scientists have a responsibility to continue to look for new stories, to find the tools we need to expand the stories we have, to include the perspectives of those we have excluded. As Haraway puts it: 'It matters what stories make worlds, what worlds make stories.'

As we have seen throughout this book, the kind of innovation we need most to tackle gender bias in medicine may not be high-tech in the conventional sense but it is definitely advanced. No technology will elevate scientists above the human challenge of storytelling; because scientists, often grasping for what appears to be immortality, will never evade that responsibility of being a human member of society.

In a sense, I think I am chasing the blue flower too. My body has always been inexplicable to me. This was problematic in the face of medical professionals or when confronted with an idea of medicine that made me feel that this was a problem of ignorance or paranoia, that sent me the subliminal messages that everything about my body should be knowable, controllable, fixable. But it is that mystery that has propelled me on in my thinking and my writing, first in my PhD, but then to find other media, like this book, that would allow me to embrace that mystery more wholeheartedly; to embrace the unknown.

It has always been the unknowns of my body that have kept me fascinated and intrigued, and now, when I feel a tension between that state of awe and what medicine purports to know about my body, when that manifests as dismissiveness of doctors or gaping voids disguised by diagrams and words about male bodies in textbooks, I see that as a limitation of science in its ability to acknowledge and accommodate the unknowns that challenge it to reinvent itself. I let that awareness that this is a systemic problem and not a problem of my own body or mind propel me on to create space for a dialogue that I hope will continue to confront science with its many contradictions and, eventually, urge it to embrace those contradictions as its engine of inspiration, as well as for social change.

One of the most important moments in my writing about my experiences in the medical system came with the responses I received to an essay I wrote for the online publication *Pulp Magazine* about my experience of having an intrauterine device (IUD, or coil) placed.[3] This particular encounter with a gynaecologist had been a strange and confounding experience that I had long dismissed as uninteresting and mundane but that had somehow manifested on the page when I'd set out to write about my own medical history. Women from across the world responded, telling me how it had resonated with them, how they too had felt the pressures of conforming to gendered stereotypes, how this had led them to silently accept uncomfortable medical procedures, to disregard their better judgement, to blame and shame themselves. These intimate and generous responses dispelled any of the lingering myths I had internalised about perfect girls who were born clean, tidy and sexy and whose vaginas accommodated tampons easily.

It seems we are all conflicted and constantly in a state of becoming the women we think we are supposed to be through our interactions with the basic and advanced technologies that surround, infuse, help and harm us. This means that by reimagining the tools we use and how they're used and what they're used for, we can begin to change what it means to be a woman, and maybe to do away with that historically loaded category all together. And perhaps that can be replaced by categories that form part of a system of medical care that is of more help to more people.

I began this book by referring to the heightened awareness people have of their bodies when they're sick or suffering – that we only really become aware of our bodies when we encounter their limitations – so people privileged by the medical system might not understand this preoccupation with their bodies. I have often been frustrated by this lack of understanding on the part of others – they made me question myself nonetheless, and sometimes wish I wasn't quite so fixated on that. But then I am reminded that experiencing our bodies' limitations also draws attention to the ways in which they enable our experience of the world. A person who has experienced the limits of their body knows themselves better because they are aware of their perspective, how it is mediated by their physiology, how their body is the set of tools that determines how they interact with the world, that frames their experience, their point of view.

Scientists can learn from this, can cultivate this sense of self-awareness, that acknowledges that our perspective is unique and valuable but never complete. Understanding more consciously what part of the world they can bring to light will allow them to mark their omissions on the map for others to explore. That's how scientists can build on the shoulders of giants, but also those of ordinary people, with equally valuable, albeit different insights. Science, as a collection of stories, will always reach for more of the truth. Open-endedness, and the ongoing struggle of coming to terms with it, are the common ground science, art and all people share.

Suzanne Anker is a Bio Artist and one of the movement's pioneers. Bio Artists cultivate the playful storytelling scientists today need to move beyond gender bias, people who boldly face the contradictions and complexities that define our experience of biology and hold a mirror up to life using life itself. Instead of using paints, these artists have in their toolkits live tissues, bacteria, living organisms and life processes.

My favourite piece of Anker's art is a series of petri dishes titled *Vanitas (in a Petri dish)*. In it, Anker seizes some of the tools, materials and methodologies of biotech researchers, along with the artistic tools of photography, symbolism and metaphor, to create seductive mini landscapes largely composed of naturally occurring materials, but also human-made – colourful flowers, insects, seeds, skeletons of small amphibians, slices of fruit, egg yolks, exoskeletons of sea urchins, drying orange peels, spiny seed pods and even small bones from the meals Anker had eaten on her way to install the exhibition.[4] Vanitas is a seventeenth-century Dutch style of still-life painting that included dead and decaying objects to remind viewers of their own mortality. Placed within and framed by the petri dishes of laboratory scientists, Anker's mini landscapes reveal the artifice of life in the biotech age and draw attention to the choices made in assembling, sustaining and prioritising lives today. In this way, Anker draws parallels between the synthetic biology creating new opportunities for intervention in the life cycle and the exploratory space of the artist's toolbox.

Anker uses the petri dishes as an artist, not as a scientist would – i.e. not as a site to grow organisms in a culture medium, not as a lens through which to prove a hypothesis through a formulaic replicability, but instead as a frame that 'cultures science'. To me, the colourful palates are a reminder that in the age of biotech, more than ever, the scientist, like the artist, chooses their palate. They choose how they render the landscape they set out to explore and with the expanding set of tools and futuristic possibilities available to them, they can more than ever choose the direction their science takes, how they wish to conduct their science, which problems they want to tackle, innovatively, whether it's from a new direction, and also, who they wish to help.

The landscapes within the petri dishes make me think about the landscapes science is creating beyond the lab, in the world beyond, and that it can choose to incorporate the unknowns and the contradictions it encounters for the betterment of that world – or to turn away from them in favour of the tried and tested blacks and whites it already knows.

This world beyond is made of connections. The connections between bodies and social and natural environments, between doctors and patients, between scientists and society. This is the space–time continuum that connects us all, and the challenge is – will always continue to be – to move through it in configurations that harness and protect the wellbeing of all. To make these connections visible, we need stories, futuristic stories that form the spaces through which scientists roam. Enter the interspecies connector created by the Bio Artist Saša Spačal.

In a piece called *Myconnect* (2013), Spačal invites visitors to participate in a dynamic and experiential form of communication between human and fungal mycelium. The human explorer enters a chamber that detects their heartbeat through sensors and then plays it back to them. This sound is then modulated by data produced through readings of the natural chemical reactions of the fungi that also occupy the chamber and these are transferred back to the human body via sound, light and haptic sensory impulses, affecting the human viewer's nervous system and heart rate so that, as the project website puts it, 'the nervous system of the person is integrated into the human-interface-mycelium feedback loop via the heartbeat'.[5] This is a cyborg machine in the form of a sensory feedback loop that reveals and expresses the subtle symbiosis between humans and their natural environment that always already exists, but is made palpable in new ways through the machine's technology.

We are connected to our environments, to other life forms, and we use our bodies and tools to interact and engage with them. We are entangled bodies, always member parts in sprawling networks. And in this complex web of interactions which we have only just begun to understand, would gender really be the prescient one? In the context of this outlandish machine, the absurdity of our human obsession with binary categorisations becomes palpable. With a plethora of undefined, unexplored, limitless feedback loops and connections that position us in the world, the challenge to science is set – start with gender differences, that's fine, but never forget that you are scratching the surface. That there are so many dimensions to explore, that you are always making a choice and, in making that choice, you decide which connections – to other people or life forms – to acknowledge, which to ignore.

It's an overwhelming thought, but we were reminded when even at the height of the pandemic, the sweeping virus revealed that true biological isolation is an impossibility – masks, walls, distance – all were ultimately futile in severing the bonds of the cells, particles, hormones, words and wires that connected us. Science – and medicine – can use its tools to better understand these connections – or it can turn a blind eye. It can expand the world of medicine to take responsibility for the social relationships that it sustains or it can continue to serve the male bodies that stand to benefit from current methods and focus. What it cannot do is disassociate itself.

The knowledge gained through science shapes and is shaped by our social world, its ideas and cures and research objectives enter a world made of power relations and scientists and medics will only reinforce the status quo if its scope and perspective do not evolve over time. Scientists have a choice in the stories they tell, as I have said during the course of this book, and the creative potential of storytelling can only serve as a model for the potential to render things anew, a prompt for science to get lost, however systematically, in a landscape that we all always already share, but one that can become more habitable to more people, the more we cultivate our shared unknowns.

Notes

Introduction

1 Photograph: Shubhangi Ganeshrao Kene/Getty Images/Science Photo Library RF.

Chapter 1

1 Public Health England. "Survey reveals women experience severe reproductive health issues". 26 June 2018. See: https://www.gov.uk/government/news/survey-reveals-women-experience-severe-reproductive-health-issues

2 Lynn, Enright. *Vagina: A Re-Education*, 2019. Allen & Unwin.

3 Jackson, G. "The endometriosis plan is good news. If funding follows". *Guardian*. 14 May 2018. See: https://www.theguardian.com/commentisfree/2018/may/14/the-endometriosis-plan-is-good-news-if-funding-follows

4 Endometriosis UK. "Endometriosis facts and figures". See: https://www.endometriosis-uk.org/endometriosis-facts-and-figures

5 Batha, E. "UK lawmakers urge action to help 1.5 mln women with endometriosis". *Reuters*. 19 October 2020. See: https://www.reuters.com/article/britain-women-health/uk-lawmakers-urge-action-to-help-1-5-mln-women-with-endometriosis-idINL8N2HA511

6 Lancucki, L., et al. "The impact of Jade Goody's diagnosis and death on the NHS Cervical Screening Programme." *Journal of medical screening*. 2012; 19(2): 89–93. doi:10.1258/jms.2012.012028.

7 *Better for women* report. "Improving the health and wellbeing of girls and women". Royal College of Obstetricians & Gynaecologists. December 2019. See: https://www.rcog.org.uk/media/h3smwohw/better-for-women-full-report.pdf.

8 Ibid.

9 Marquez, P. V. "Healthy women are the cornerstone of healthy societies". World Bank Blogs. 12 January 2017. See: https://blogs.worldbank.org/health/healthy-women-are-cornerstone-healthy-societies

Chapter 2

1 A study released in 2020 confirmed that the HPV vaccine substantially reduces invasive cervical cancer risk. The researchers followed over 1.5 million girls and women in Sweden for up to eleven years and found that the risk of cervical cancer by age thirty was 65% lower in vaccinated women compared with unvaccinated women. Public Health England released a report in 2018, 10 years after the vaccination programme was introduced in the UK, showing that there was an 86% reduction in HPV types 16/18 in sixteen-to-twenty-one-year-old women. While there remains work to be done in low- and middle-income countries to scale up vaccinations, high-income countries are on track to eliminate the virus.

2 Sandall, J., Soltani, H., Gates, S., Shennan, A. & Devane, D. "Midwife-led continuity models of care compared with other models of care for women during pregnancy, birth and early parenting". Cochrane. 28 April 2016. See: https://www.cochrane.org/CD004667/PREG_midwife-led-continuity-models-care-compared-other-models-care-women-during-pregnancy-birth-and-early

3 Five Year Forward View. "Implementing Better Births: Continuity of Carer". NHS. December 2017. See: https://www.england.nhs.uk/wp-content/uploads/2017/12/implementing-better-births.pdf

4 Sanders, J., Hunter, B. & Warren, L. "A wall of information?

Exploring the public health component of maternity care in England". *Midwifery*. March 2016. 34:253–260. See: https://doi.org/10.1016/j.midw.2015.10.013

5 Five Year Forward View. "Implementing Better Births: Continuity of Carer".

6 While governments are increasingly investing in long COVID research, this fades in comparison to the (largely, publicly funded) government investments into the development of vaccines. The UK government, for example, announced that it would invest £18.5 million into long COVID research in 2021, in comparison to the £38.6 million that by 2021 had gone into the Oxford/AstraZeneca vaccines alone. See: https://www.gov.uk/government/news/185-million-to-tackle-long-covid-through-research; https://www.theguardian.com/science/2021/apr/15/oxfordastrazeneca-covid-vaccine-research-was-97-publicly-funded; https://www.medrxiv.org/content/10.1101/2021.04.08.21255103v1.full.pdf; https://covid19.trackvaccines.org/agency/who/

7 A 2020 study, conducted by RAND Europe and commissioned by the UK Clinical Research Collaboration and funded by NIHR and Wellcome Trust, in this way analysed current funding for pregnancy-related research in the UK, and prioritised key issues in the field by combining the views of researchers, healthcare professionals and the public. In their survey of over 600 participants, mental health problems during and after pregnancy ranked as the top priority areas across stakeholders, after which came issues around medication, stillbirth and breastfeeding. Mental health, then, is recognised as a priority area by all those most directly concerned with ensuring healthy pregnancies.

8 NICE. "Antenatal and postnatal mental health: clinical management and service guidance". Updated 11 February 2020. See: https://www.nice.org.uk/guidance/cg192/chapter/introduction

9 For example, guidelines published in 2015 estimate that 85% of localities do not have specialist perinatal mental health services providing care to the level recommended in practice guidelines.

10 A Dutch study showed that only one-third of all men and only 20% of men over the age of 70 with significant erectile dysfunction had major psychological concerns. Furthermore, in sexually active men, 17–28% had no normal erections, indicating that full erectile function is not essential for sexual functioning. Blanker, M. H., et al. "Erectile and ejaculatory dysfunction in a community-based sample of men 50 to 78 years old: Prevalence, concern, and relation to sexual activity". *Urology*. 2001. 57:763–768.

Chapter 3

1 Gunter, J. "Dear Gwyneth Paltrow, I'm a GYN and your vaginal jade eggs are a bad idea". 17 January 2017. See: https://drjengunter.com/2017/01/17/dear-gwyneth-paltrow-im-a-gyn-and-your-vaginal-jade-eggs-are-a-bad-idea/

2 Brodesser-Akner, T. "How Goop's haters made Gwyneth Paltrow's company worth $250 million". *New York Times Magazine*. 25 July 2018. See: https://www.nytimes.com/2018/07/25/magazine/big-business-gwyneth-paltrow-wellness.html

3 Sack, Georgeann. *Kegels Are Not Going to Fix This*, 2020. Afferent, LLC.

4 Shah, S., M., Sultan, A. H. & Thakar, R. "The history and evolution of pessaries for pelvic organ prolapse". *International Urogynecology Journal*. 2005; 17:170–175. See: https://link.springer.com/article/10.1007/s00192-005-1313-6. Green, M. H., ed. *The Trotula: An English translation of the medieval compendium of women's medicine*. University of Pennsylvania Press, 2013. Frymer-Kensky, T. "The Strange Case of the Suspected Sotah", in "Women in the Hebrew Bible", ed. Bach (1999, New York and London: Routledge, pages 463–474).

5 Shah, S., et al. "The history and evolution of pessaries . . ."

6 Abhyankar, P., Uny, I., Semple, K., et al. "Women's experiences of receiving care for pelvic organ prolapse: a qualitative study". *BMC Women's Health*. 2019; 19(45).

Chapter 4

1 The Anatomy Lesson of Dr. Nicolaes Tulp, Rembrandt van Rijn. See:
https://commons.wikimedia.org/wiki/Category:The_Anatomy_
Lesson_of_Dr._Nicolaes_Tulp#/media/File:Rembrandt_-_The_
Anatomy_Lecture_of_Dr._Nicolaes_Tulp_-_WGA19139.jpg

2 Sebald, W. G. *The Rings of Saturn*, 1995. London: New Directions
Books.

3 Masters, W. H. and Johnson, V. E. *Human Sexual Response*, 1966.
Boston: Little Brown & Co.

4 Chivers, M. L., Rieger, G., Latty, E., et al. "A Sex Difference in the
Specificity of Sexual Arousal". *Psychological Science*. 2004; 15(11):
736–744. See: https://doi.org/10.1111/j.0956-7976.2004.00750.

5 Katherine, Angel. *Tomorrow Sex Will Be Good Again*, 2021. Verso.

6 Gilliland, Amy. "Women's experiences of female ejaculation".
Sexuality & Culture. 2009; 13(3).

7 Bering, Jesse. "Female ejaculation: the long road to non-discovery".
17 June 2011. See: https://blogs.scientificamerican.com/bering-in-
mind/female-ejaculation-the-long-road-to-non-discovery

8 Whitney, Ev'Yan. "An Open Letter to Women Who Squirt".
26 January 2022. See: https://evyanwhitney.com/letter-to-
squirters/?fbclid=IwAR2YMUT_zsyjlYOTEPl9mykEdwe
SuQpAnLIeya-KBWpuhsC6Hz_8HkErxX4

9 Ligon, Z. "What Learning to Squirt Taught Me About My
Body". *Refinery 29*. 1 February 2016. See: https://www.refin-
ery29.com/en-us/what-is-squirting

10 Wimpissinger, F., & Springer, C., et al. "International online
survey: female ejaculation has a positive impact on women's and
their partners' sexual lives". *Sexual Medicine*. 2013; 112(2).

11 Bell, Shannon. *Whore Carnival* (New York: Autonomedia,
1995).

Chapter 5

1 Lacquer, Thomas. *Making Sex: Body and Gender from the Greeks to Freud*. Harvard University Press, 1992.

2 Oudshoorn, N. *Beyond the Natural Body*. London: Routledge, 1994.

3 Grover, N. "Not accounting for sex differences in Covid research could be deadly". *Guardian*. 25 September 2020. See: https://www.theguardian.com/science/2020/sep/25/not-accounting-for-sex-differences-in-covid-research-can-be-deadly

4 Nehm, R. H. & Young, R. "'Sex Hormones' in Secondary School Biology Textbooks". *Science & Education*. 2008; 17: 1175–1190. See: https://doi.org/10.1007/s11191-008-9137-7

5 Bertelloni, S., Meriggioloa, M. C., Dati, E., et al. "Bone Mineral Density in Women Living with Complete Androgen Insensitivity Syndrome and Intact Testes or Removed Gonads". *Sexual Development*. 2017; 11(4). See also: Soule, S. G., et al. "Osteopenia as a feature of the androgen insensitivity syndrome". *Clin. Endocrinol*. 43, 6 (1995): 671–675; *Int. J. Mol. Sci*. 22, 3 (2021): 1264; See: https://doi.org/10.3390/ijms22031264 See also: https://doi.org/10.1159/000477599 See also:10.1210/jendso/bvab048.1584;

6 Dohnert, U., Wunsch, L. & Hiort, O. "Gonadectomy in Complete Androgen Insensitivity Syndrome: Why and When?". *Sexual Development*. 2017; 11:4. See: https://doi.org/10.1159/000478082

7 Birnbaum, W., Marshall, L., et al. "Oestrogen versus androgen in hormone-replacement therapy for complete androgen insensitivity syndrome: a multicentre, randomised, double-dummy, double-blind crossover trial". *The Lancet: Diabetes & Endocrinology*. 2018; 6(10): 771–780. See: https://doi.org/10.1016/S2213-8587(18)30197-9

8 The World Health Organization (WHO) defines QOL as 'an individual's perception of their position in life in context of the culture and value systems in which they live, and in relation to their goals, expectations, standards and concerns'.

9 Rapp, Marion, et al. "Quality of life in adults with disorders/differences of sex development (DSD) compared to country specific reference populations". 2018. See: https://www.dsd-life.eu/fileadmin/websites/dsd-life/images/Flyer/Quality_of_life_Final.pdf

10 Preciado, Paul B. *Can the Monster Speak?*, trans. Frank Wynne, pp. 19–20 (Fitzcarraldo Editions, 2021).

11 Guilbert, K. "Surgery and sterilizations scrapped in Malta's benchmark LGBTI law". *Reuters*. 1 April 2015. See: https://www.reuters.com/article/us-gay-rights-malta-idUSKBN0MS4ZE20150401

12 Human Rights for Hermaphrodites Too!. "Submission for OHCHR Study on Youth and Human Rights (HRC39)". StopIGM.org. See: https://www.ohchr.org/Documents/Issues/Youth/StopIGM.pdf

13 "Intersex Genital Mutilations: Human Rights Violations of Children with Variations of Reproductive Anatomy". CAT UK NGO Report, 2019. See: https://tbinternet.ohchr.org/Treaties/CAT/Shared%20Documents/GBR/INT_CAT_CSS_GBR_34414_E.pdf

Part 2

1 Kaminsky, L. The Health Gap. "The case for renaming women's body parts". *BBC Future*. 4 June 2018. See: https://www.bbc.com/future/article/20180531-how-womens-body-parts-have-been-named-after-men

Chapter 6

1 Sorge, R. E., et al. "Spinal Cord Toll-Like Receptor 4 Mediates Inflammatory and Neuropathic Hypersensitivity in Male But Not Female Mice". *Journal of Neuroscience*. 2011; 31: 15450–15454. See: https://doi.org/10.1523/JNEUROSCI.3859-11.2011

2 Sorge, R. E., et al. "Different immune cells mediate mechanical pain hypersensitivity in male and female mice". *Nat Neurosci*. 2015; 18: 1081–1083. See: https://pubmed.ncbi.nlm.nih.gov/26120961/

3 Mogil, J. S. & Chanda, M. L. "The case for the inclusion of female subjects in basic science studies of pain". *Pain*. 2005; 117:1–5; Prendergast, B. J., Onishi, K. G. & Zucker, I. "Female mice liberated for inclusion in neuroscience and biomedical research". *Neurosci. Biobehav. Rev.* 2014; 40: 1–5; Itoh, Y. & Arnold, A. P. "Are females more variable than males in gene expression? Meta-analysis of microarray datasets". *Biol. Sex. Diff.* 2015; 6, 18; Becker, J. B., Prendergast, B. J. & Liang, J. W. "Female rats are not more variable than male rats: a meta-analysis of neuroscience studies". *Biol. Sex. Diff.* 2016; 7, 34.

4 Beery, A. K. & Zucker, I. "Sex bias in neuroscience and biomedical research". *Neurosci. Biobehav. Rev.* 2010; 35: 565–572; Klein, S. & Flanagan, K. "Sex differences in immune responses". *Nat. Rev. Immunol.* 2016; 16: 626–638. See: https://doi.org/10.1038/nri.2016.90

5 Mogil, J. S. "Qualitative sex differences in pain processing: emerging evidence of a biased literature". *Nature Reviews Neuroscience*. 2020; 21: 353–365. See: https://doi.org/10.1038/s41583-020-0310-6

6 Mogil, J. S. & Chanda, M. L. "The case for the inclusion of female subjects in basic science studies of pain". *Pain*. 2005; 117: 1–5. See: https://pubmed.ncbi.nlm.nih.gov/16098670/

7 Mogil, J. S. "Qualitative sex differences in pain processing . . ."

8 Quoting the 12th-century Neo-Platonist scholar Bernard of Chartres.

9 Sorge, R. E., et al. "Different immune cells mediate mechanical pain . . ." See: https://doi.org/10.1038/nn.4053

10 Sorge, R. E., et al. "Olfactory exposure to males, including men, causes stress and related analgesia in rodents". *Nature Methods*. 2014; 11: 629–632. See: https://doi.org/10.1038/nmeth.2935

11 Brown, K. J. & Grunberg, N. E. "Effects of housing on male and female rats: crowding stresses males but calms females". *Physiol. Behav.* 1995; 58: 1085–1089. See: https://psycnet.apa.org/record/1996-25742-001

12 Song, Z., et al. "High-fat diet exacerbates postoperative pain and inflammation in a sex-dependent manner". *Pain*. 2018; 159: 1731–1741. See: https://pubmed.ncbi.nlm.nih.gov/29708941/

13 Levine, F. M. & De Simone, L. L. "The effects of experimenter gender on pain report in male and female subjects". *Pain*. 1991; 44: 69–72. See: https://pubmed.ncbi.nlm.nih.gov/2038491/

14 Essick, G., et al. "Site-dependent and subject-related variations in perioral thermal sensitivity". *Somatosens. Mot. Res.* 2004; 21: 159–175; Otto, M. W. & Dougher, M. J. "Sex differences and personality factors in responsivity to pain." *Percept. Mot. Skills*. 1985; 61: 383–390.

15 Kallai, I., Barke, A. & Voss, U. "The effects of experimenter characteristics on pain reports in women and men". *Pain*. 2004; 112: 142–147.

16 Stanke, K. M. & Ivanec, D. "Pain threshold – measure of pain sensitivity or social behavior?". *Psihologija*. 2016; 49: 37–50.

17 Vigil, J. M., Rowell, L. N., Alcocvk, J. & Maestes, R. "Laboratory personnel gender and cold pressor apparatus affect subjective pain reports". *Pain. Res. Manag.* 2014; 19: e13–e18.

18 Edwards, R., Eccleston, C. & Keogh, E. "Observer influences on pain: an experimental series examining same-sex and opposite-sex friends, strangers, and romantic partners". *Pain*. 2017; 158: 846–855.

19 Pelletier, R., et al. "Sex-related differences in access to care among patients with premature acute coronary syndrome". *CMAJ*. 2014; 186(7): 497–504. See: https://doi.org/10.1503/cmaj.131450

20 Chen, E. H., Shofer, F. S., Anthony, J. D., et al. "Gender disparity in analgesic treatment of emergency department patients with acute abdominal pain". *Academic Emergency Medicine*. 2008; 15(5): 414–418. See: https://doi.org/10.1111/j.1553-2712.2008.00100.x

21 Hoffmann, D. E. & Tarzian, A. J. "The Girl Who Cried Pain: A Bias Against Women in the Treatment of Pain". *SSRN*. 2001. See: http://dx.doi.org/10.2139/ssrn.383803

22 Robertson, J. "Waiting Time at the Emergency Department from a Gender Equality Perspective". *University of Gothenburg: Programme in Medicine*. 2014. See: https://gupea.ub.gu.se/bitstream/2077/39196/1/gupea_2077_39196_1.pdf

23 Aloisi, A. M., et al. "Cross-sex hormone administration changes

pain in transsexual women and men". *Pain*. 2007; 132: S60–S67. See: https://pubmed.ncbi.nlm.nih.gov/17379410/

24 Rosen, S. F., et al. "T-Cell Mediation of Pregnancy Analgesia Affecting Chronic Pain in Mice". *J. Neurosci*. 2017; 37: 9819–9827. See: https://www.jneurosci.org/content/37/41/9819

25 Hoffman, K. M., Trawalter, S., Axt, J. R. & Oliver, M. N. "Racial bias in pain assessment and treatment recommendations, and false beliefs about biological differences between Blacks and whites". *Proc Natl Acad Sci USA*. 2016; 113: 4296–4301.

26 Meghani, S. H., Byun, E. & Gallagher, R. M. "Time to take stock: a meta-analysis and systematic review of analgesic treatment disparities for pain in the United States." *Pain Med*. 2012; 13: 150–174.

27 Hoffman, K., et al. "Racial bias in pain . . ." See: https://doi.org/10.1073/pnas.1516047113 See also: https://www.rcog.org.uk/globalassets/documents/news/position-statements/racial-disparities-womens-healthcare-march-2020.pdf

28 Oxford Population Health NPEU. "MBRRACE-UK: Mothers and Babies: Reducing Risk through audits and Confidential Enquiries across the UK". See: https://www.npeu.ox.ac.uk/mbrrace-uk

29 Sakala, Carol, et al. "Listening to Mothers in California: A Population-Based Survey of Women's Childbearing Experiences, Full Survey Report". Washington: National Partnership for Women of Families, 2018. See: https://www.chcf.org/wp-content/uploads/2018/09/ListeningMothersCAFullSurveyReport2018.pdf?utm_source=National%20Partnership&utm_medium=PDF_Link&utm_campaign=Listening%20to%20Mothers; Martin, Nina and Montagne, Renee. "Lost Mothers: Nothing Protects Black Women From Dying in Pregnancy and Childbirth." *ProPublica*, 7 December 2017. See: https://www.propublica.org/article/nothing-protects-black-women-from-dying-in-pregnancy-and-childbirth See also: https://doi.org/10.1093/jpepsy/jsy104

Chapter 7

1 Prasad, A., Lerman, A. & Rihal, C. S. "Apical ballooning syndrome (Tako-Tsubo or stress cardiomyopathy): a mimic of acute myocardial infarction". *Am Heart J.* 2008; 155: 408–417; Vidi, V., et al. "Clinical characteristics of Tako-Tsubo cardiomyopathy." *Am J. Cardiol.* 2009; 104: 578–582.

2 Pattisapu, V. K., Hao, H., Liu, Y., et al. "Sex- and Age-Based Temporal Trends in Takotsubo Syndrome Incidence in the United States". *Am Heart J.* 2012; 10(20). See: https://doi.org/10.1161/JAHA.120.019583

3 Summers, M. R., Lennon, R. J. & Prasad, A. "Pre-morbid psychiatric and cardiovascular diseases in apical ballooning syndrome (Tako-Tsubo/stress-induced cardiomyopathy)." *J. Am Coll Cardiol.* 2010; 55: 700–701.

4 Das, S. "It's hysteria, not a heart attack, GP app Babylon tells women". *The Times.* 13 October 2019. See: https://www.thetimes.co.uk/article/its-hysteria-not-a-heart-attack-gp-app-tells-women-gm2vxbrqk

5 Rozanski, A., et al. "The epidemiology, pathophysiology and management of psychosocial risk factors in cardiac practice". *J Am Coll Cardiol.* 2005; 45: 637–651.

6 Low, C. A., Thurston, R. C. & Matthews, K. A. "Psychosocial factors in the development of heart disease in women: current research and future directions." *Psychosom Med.* 72 (2010): 842–854.

7 Benjamin, E. J., et al. "Heart Disease and Stroke Statistics–2018 Update: A report from the American Heart Association". 2018; 137:367–e492. See: https://doi.org/10.1161/CIR.0000000000000558; Kalinowski, J., Taylor, J. Y. & Spruill, T. M. "Why Are Young Black Women at High Risk for Cardiovascular Disease?". *Circulation.* 2019; 139: 1003–1004. See: https://doi.org/10.1161/CIRCULATIONAHA.118.037689

8 Smilowitz, N. R., Maduro, G. A., Lobach, I. V., et al. "Adverse Trends in Ischemic Heart Disease Mortality among Young New Yorkers, Particularly Young Black Women". *PLoS ONE.* 2016;

11(2): e0149015. See: https://doi.org/10.1371/journal.pone.0149015

9 Orth-Gomer, K. & Leineweber, C. "Multiple stressors and coronary disease in women. The Stockholm female coronary risk study". *Biol Psychol.* 2005; 69: 57–66.

10 Konst, R. E., et al. "Different cardiovascular risk factors and psychosocial burden in symptomatic women with and without obstructive coronary artery disease". *Eur. J. Prev. Cardiol.* 2019; 26: 657–659; Vaccarino, V., et al. "Mental stress-induced-myocardial ischemia in young patients with recent myocardial infarction: sex differences and mechanisms". *Circulation.* 2018; 137: 794–805.

11 Maas, A. H. E. M., van der Schouw, Y. T., Regitz-Zagrosek, V., et al. "Red alert for women's heart: the urgent need for more research and knowledge on cardiovascular disease in women: Proceedings of the Workshop held in Brussels on Gender Differences in Cardiovascular disease". *Eur. Heart Journal.* 2010; 32(11): 1362–1368. See: https://doi.org/10.1093/eurheartj/ehr048

12 Jones, L. "Architecture of the heart different between women and men and with age". BHF. 31 August 2020. See: https://www.bhf.org.uk/what-we-do/news-from-the-bhf/news-archive/2020/august/esc-heart-shape-structure-men-women-qmul

13 Ji, H., Niiranen, T. J., Rader, F., et al. "Sex Differences in Blood Pressure Associations with Cardiovascular Outcomes". *Circulation.* 2021;143(7):761–763.See:https://doi.org/10.1161/CIRCULATIONAHA.120.049360

14 Towfighi, A., Zheng, L. & Ovbiagele, B. "Sex-specific trends in midlife coronary heart disease risk and prevalence". *Arch. Intern. Med.* 2009; 169: 1762–1766.

15 Stress in America. "Stress and Gender". *American Psychological Association.* 2010. See: https://www.apa.org/news/press/releases/stress/2010/gender-stress.pdf

16 Gonsalves, C. A., McGannon, K. R., Schinke, R. J. & Pegoraro, A. "Mass media narratives of women's cardiovascular disease: a

qualitative meta-synthesis". *Health Psychology Review*. 2017; 11(2): 174–178. See: https://doi.org/10.1080/17437199.2017.1281750

17 Mgbako, O. U., Ha, Y. P., Ranard, B. L., et al. "Defibrillation in the movies: A missed opportunity for public health education". *Resuscitation*. 2014; 85(12): 1795–1798. See: https://doi.org/ 10.1016/j.resuscitation.2014.09.005

18 Mosca, L., Ferris, A., Fabunmi, R., et al. "Tracking Women's Awareness of Heart Disease". *Circulation*. 2004; 109: 573–579. See: https://www.ahajournals.org/doi/10.1161/01.CIR.0000115222. 69428.C9

19 Berry, T. R., Stearns. J. A., Courneya, K. S., et al. "Women's perception of heart disease and breast cancer and the association with media representations of the diseases". *Journal of Public Health*. 2016; 38(4): e496–e503. See: https://doi.org/10.1093/pubmed/ fdv177

20 Radboud U. M. C. "Pregnancy complications and early meno-pause affect cardiovascular disease in women". 9 February 2021. See: https://www.radboudumc.nl/en/news/2021/pregnancy-complications-and-early-menopause-affect-cardiovascular-disease -in-women

21 Maas, A. H. E. M., Rosano, G., Cifkova, R., et al. "Cardiovascular health after menopause transition, pregnancy disorders, and other gynaecologic conditions: a consensus document from European cardiologists, gynaecologists, and endocrinologists". *European Heart Journal*. 2021; 42(10): 967–984. See: https://doi.org/ 10.1093/eurheartj/ehaa1044

22 Manson, J. E., et al. "Estrogen plus progestin and the risk of coro-nary heart disease". *New England Journal of Medicine*. 2003; 349: 523–534.

23 Gast, G.C.M., et al. "Menopausal complaints are associated with cardiovascular risk factors". *Hypertension*. 2008; 51: 1492–1498; Gast, G.C.M., et al. "Vasomotor menopausal symptoms are asso-ciated with increased risk of coronary heart disease". *Menopause*. 2011; 18: 146–151.

24 Mikkola, T. S. & Clarkson, T. B. "Estrogen replacement therapy,

atherosclerosis and vascular function". *Cardiovasc. Res.* 2002; 53: 605–619.

25 Bellamy, L., Casas, J. P., Hingorani, A. D. & Williams, D. J. "Preeclampsia and risk of cardio-vascular disease and cancer later in life: systematic review and meta-analysis". *BMJ.* 2007; 335: 974–983; Magnussen, E. B., Vatten, L. J., Smith, G. D. & Romundstad, P. R. "Hypertensive disorders in pregnancy and subsequently measured cardiovascular risk factors". *Obstet. Gynaecol.* 2009; 114: 961–970.

26 McDonald, S. D., et al. "Cardiovascular sequelae of preeclampsia/eclampsia: a systematic review and meta-analysis". *Am Heart J.* 2008; 156: 918–930.

27 Drost, J. T., Maas, A. H., van Eyck J. & van der Schouw Y. T. "Preeclampsia as a female-specific risk factor for chronic hypertension". *Maturitas.* 2010; 67: 321–326.

28 Maas, Angela. *A Woman's Heart* (Hachette UK, 2020).

29 Nota, N. M., et al. "Occurrence of acute cardiovascular events in transgender individuals receiving hormone therapy". *Circulation.* 2019; 139: 1461–1462.

30 Getahun, D., et al. "Cross-sex hormones and acute cardiovascular events in transgender persons: a cohort study". *Ann. Intern. Med.* 2018; 169: 205–213.

31 Nota, N. M., et al. "Occurrence of acute cardiovascular events in transgender individuals receiving hormone therapy". *Circulation.* 2019; 139: 1461–1462.

32 Mieres, J. H., et al. "Role of Noninvasive Testing in the Clinical Evaluation of Women with Suspected Coronary Artery Disease: Consensus Statement from the Cardiac Imaging Committee, Council on Clinical Cardiology, and the Cardiovascular Imaging and Intervention Committee, Council on Cardiovascular Radiology and Intervention, American Heart Association". *Circulation.* 2005; 111: 682–696; Stangl, V., Witzel, V., Baumann, G. & Stangl, K. "Current diagnostic concepts to detect coronary artery disease in women". *Eur. Heart J.* 2008; 29: 707–717; Wenger, N. K., Shaw, L. J. & Vaccarino, V. "Coronary heart

disease in women: update 2008". *Clin. Pharmacol. Ther.* 2008; 83: 37–51.

33 Jacobs, A. K. "Coronary intervention in 2009. Are women no different than men?". *Circ. Cardiovasc. Intervent.* 2009; 2: 69–78.

34 Gulati, M., et al. "Adverse cardiovascular outcomes in women with nonobstructive coronary artery disease. A report from the Women's Ischemia Syndrome Evaluation Study and the St James Women Take Heart Project". *Arch. Intern. Med.* 2009; 169: 843–850; Arant, C. B. "Multimarker approach predicts adverse cardiovascular events in women evaluated for suspected ischemia: a report from the NHLBI –sponsored WISE-study". *Clin. Cardiol.* 2009; 32: 244–250.

35 Pepine, C. J., et al. "Coronary microvascular reactivity to adenosine predicts adverse outcome in women evaluated for suspected ischemia. Results from the National Heart, Lung and Blood Institute WISE (Women's Ischemia Syndrome Evaluation) Study". *J. Am. Coll. Cardiol.* 2010; 55: 2825–2832.

36 Kruk, M., et al. "Intravascular ultrasonic study of gender differences in ruptured coronary plaque morphology and its associated clinical presentation". *Am. J. Cardiol.* 2007; 100: 185–189.

Chapter 8

1 Haas, R., Watson, J., Buonasera, T., et al. "Female hunters of the early Americas". *Science Advances.* 2020; 6(45): 245–361. See: https://doi.org/10.1126/sciadv.abd0310

2 Anne Fausto-Sterling. "The Bare Bones of Sex: Part 1 – Sex and Gender." *Signs.* 2005; 30(2). See: https://www.jstor.org/stable/10.1086/424932

3 Ibid.

4 De Martinis, M., Sirufo, M. M., Polsinelli, M., et al. "Gender Differences in Osteoporosis: A Single-Centre Observational Study". *World J Mens Health.* 2021; 39(4):750–759. See: https://doi.org/10.5534/wjmh.200099

5 Alswat, K. "Gender Disparities in Osteoporosis". *Journal of Clinical Medicine Research.* 2017; 9(5): 382–387. See: https://doi.org/10.14740/jocmr2970w

6 Fugh-Berman, A., Pearson, C. K., Allina, A., Zones, J., Worcester, N. & Whatley, M. 2002 in "The Bare Bones of Sex: Part 1 – Sex and Gender" by Fausto-Sterling.

7 Anne Fausto-Sterling. "The Bare Bones of Sex: Part 1 – Sex and Gender." *Signs*. 2005; 30(2). https://www.jstor.org/stable/10.1086/424932

8 Fugh-Berman, A., Pearson, C. K., Allina, A., Zones, J., Worcester, N. & Whatley, M. 2002 in "The Bare Bones of Sex: Part 1 – Sex and Gender" by Fausto-Sterling.

9 Meunier, Pierre J. 1988. "Assessment of Bone Turnover by Historimorphometry". *Osteoporosis: Etiology, Diagnosis, and Management*, ed. B. Lawrence Riggs and L. Joseph Melton III, 317–332. New York: Raven.

10 Zanchetta, J. R., Plotkin, H. & Alvarez Filgueira, M. L. "Bone Mass in Children: Normative Values for the 2–20-Year-Old Population". *Bone*. 1995; 16: S393–S399.

11 van Staa T. P. "Epidemiology of fractures in England and Wales". *Bone*. 2001; 29: 517–522; NIH Consensus Statement Online. 17, no. 1 (2000): 1–36.

12 Taha, Wael., et al. "Reduced Spinal Bone Mineral Density in Adolescents of an Ultra-Orthodox Jewish Community in Brooklyn". *Pediatrics*. 2001; 107: e79–e85. In Fausto-Sterling, "The Bare Bones of Sex".

13 Nesby-O'Dell, S., et al. "Hypovitaminosis D Prevalence and Determinants Among African American and White Women of Reproductive Age: Third National Health and Nutrition Examination Survey, 1988–1994". *American Journal of Clinical Nutrition*. 2002; 76(1): 187–192.

14 This updated statistics build on Fausto-Sterling's proposed paradigm for health and disease, which draws on the contributions of geographic ancestry, individual lifecycle experience, race, and gender. See: Fausto-Sterling, A. (2008). The Bare Bones of Race. Social Studies of Science, 38(5), 657–694. https://doi.org/10.1177/0306312708091925.

15 Fausto-Sterling, A. (2008). The Bare Bones of Race. Social

Studies of Science, 38(5), 657–694. https://doi.org/10.1177/03063 12708091925

16 Vieth, R. "Effects of Vitamin D on Bone and Natural Selection of Skin Color: How much Vitamin D Nutrition are we Talking About?". *Bone Loss and Osteoporosis: An Anthropological Perspective*, ed. S. Agarwal & S. D. Stout, 139–154 (New York: Kluwer Academic/Plenum Publishers, 2003).

17 Shaw, N. J. & Pal, B. R. "Vitamin D Deficiency in UK Asian Families: Activating a New Concern". *Archives of Disease in Childhood*. 2002: 86(3): 147–149; Meyer, H. E. E., et al. "Vitamin D Deficiency and Secondary Hyperparathyroidism and the Association with Bone Mineral Density in Persons with Pakistani and Norwegian Background Living in Oslo, Norway, The Oslo Health Study". *Bone*. 35(2): 412–417.

18 Roberts, M. "Coronavirus: Should I start taking vitamin D?". *BBC News*. See: https://www.bbc.co.uk/news/health-52371688

19 The Human Genome Project was an international scientific research project, funded by the US government, and launched in 1990, that aimed to identify, map and sequence all of the genes of the human genome. The project was declared complete in 2003, when scientists had accounted for about 85% of the genome. By 2022, scientists had addressed the final gaps. Further information available here: https://web.ornl.gov/sci/techresources/Human_ Genome/project/index.shtml

20 See for example: Opotowsky, Alexander R. & Bilezikian, John P. "Racial Differences in the Effect of Early Milk Consumption on Peak and Postmenopausal Bone Mineral Density". *Journal of Bone and Mineral Research*. 2003; 18(11): 1978–1988; Taaffe, D. R., et al. "Lower Extremity Physical Performance and Hip Bone Mineral Density in Elderly Black and White Men and Women: Cross-sectional Associations in the Health AB" (2003).

21 Waddington, C. H. *Organisers and Genes* (Cambridge: Cambridge University Press, 1940).

22 Waddington, C. H. *Strategy of the Genes* (Oxon and New York: Routledge, 1957). In Susan Squier, *Epigenetic Landscapes*, 2017.

Chapter 9

1 Rebecca Skloot's *The Immortal Life of Henrietta Lacks* (2010) gives a seminal and thorough account of Henrietta's life and the life of her cells.

2 Smith, R. P. "Famed for 'Immortal' Cells, Henrietta Lacks is Immortalized in Portraiture". *Smithsonian Magazine*. 15 May 2018. See: https://www.smithsonianmag.com/smithsonian-institution/famed-immortal-cells-henrietta-lacks-immortalized-portraiture-180969085/

3 Callaway, E. "Deal done over HeLa cell line". *Nature*. 2013; 500: 132–133. See: https://www.nature.com/news/deal-done-over-hela-cell-line-1.13511

4 NIH. "Significant Research advances Enabled by HeLa Cells". See: https://osp.od.nih.gov/scientific-sharing/hela-cells-timeline/#:~:text=Scientists%20use%20HeLa%20cells%20to%20discover%20how%20the%20presence%20of,the%20first%20anti%2Dcancer%20vaccines.

5 Hudson, K. & Collins, F. "Family matters". *Nature*. 2013; 500: 141–142. See: https://doi.org/10.1038/500141a

6 Melinda Cooper and Catherine Waldby. *Clinical Labor: Tissue Donors and Research Subjects in the Global Bioeconomy* (Durham: Duke University Press, 2014).

7 Ibid.

8 Boshart, M., et al. "A new type of papillomavirus DNA, its presence in genital cancer biopsies and in cell lines derived from cervical cancer". *The EMBO Journal*. 1984; 3(5): 1151–1157.

9 World Health Organization. "World Health Assembly adopts global strategy to accelerate cervical cancer elimination". Departmental news. 19 August 2020. See: https://www.who.int/news/item/19-08-2020-world-health-assembly-adopts-global-strategy-to-accelerate-cervical-cancer-elimination

10 Burchell, A. N. "Chapter 6: epidemiology and transmission dynamics of genital HPV infection". *Vaccine*. 2006; 24.

11 Chesson, H. W. "The estimated lifetime probability of acquiring

human papillomavirus in the United States". *Sex. Transm. Dis.* 2014; 41(11): 660–664.

12 Giuliano, A. R. "EUROGIN 2014 roadmap: differences in human papillomavirus infection natural history, transmission and human papillomavirus–related cancer incidence by gender and anatomic site of infection". *Int. J. Cancer.* 2014; 136(12): 2752–2760. See: https://pubmed.ncbi.nlm.nih.gov/25043222/

13 Oudshoorn, N. *The Male Pill: a Biography of a Technology in the Making* (Durham: Duke University Press, 2003). Designing technology and masculinity: challenging the invisibility of male reproductive bodies in scientific medicine, pp. 1–18; de Melo-Martin I. "The promise of the human papillomavirus vaccine does not confer immunity against ethical reflection." *Oncologist* 11, no. 4 (2006): 393–396.

14 Westbrook, L. & Fourie, I. "A feminist information engagement framework for gynecological cancer patients". *J. Doc.* 2015; 71(4): 752–774.

15 Davis, J. L., Buchanan, K. L., Katz, R. V. & Green, B. L. "Gender differences in cancer screening beliefs, behaviors, and willingness to participate: implications for health promotion." *Am J Mens Health.* 2012; 6(3): 211–217. doi: 10.1177/1557988311425853.

16 Ibid.

17 Melinda Cooper and Catherine Waldby. *Clinical Labor: Tissue Donors and Research Subjects in the Global Bioeconomy* (Durham: Duke University Press, 2014).

18 Beskow, L. M. "Lessons from HeLa Cells: The Ethics and Policy of Biospecimens". *Annual Review of Genomics and Human Genetics.* 2016; 17:395–417. See: https://doi.org/10.1146/annurev-genom-083115-022536

19 Daley, E. M., Vamos, C. A., Thompson, E. L., et al. "The feminization of HPV; How science, politics, economics and gender norms shaped U.S. HPV vaccine implementation". *Papillomavirus Research.* 2017; 3:142–148. See: https://doi.org/10.1016/j.pvr.2017.04.004

Chapter 10

1 Martin, E. "The Egg and the Sperm: How Science Has Constructed a Romance Based on Stereotypical Male-Female Roles". *Chicago Journals*. 1991; 16(3): 485–501. See: https://web.stanford.edu/~eckert/PDF/Martin1991.pdf

2 Sanders, R. "Preventing sperm's 'power kick' could be key to unisex contraceptive". Berkeley Research. 17 March 2016. See: https://vcresearch.berkeley.edu/news/preventing-sperms-power-kick-could-be-key-unisex-contraceptive

3 Fitzpatrick, J. L., Willis, C., Devigili, A., et al. "Chemical signals from eggs facilitate cryptic female choice in humans". *Proceedings of the Royal Society of Biological Sciences*. 2020; 287(1928): 20200805. See: https://doi.org/10.1098/rspb.2020.0805

4 Dow, K. "Looking into the Test Tube: The Birth of IVF on British Television". *Medical History*. 2019; 63(2): 189–208. See: doi:10.1017/mdh.2019.6

Chapter 11

1 Weiss, S. "What is FemTech? 5 things to know about the new industry". *Bustle*. 16 April 2018. See: https://www.bustle.com/p/what-is-femtech-5-things-to-know-about-the-new-industry-8792289

2 Frost & Sullivan. "The COVID-19 Pandemic and a Rising Focus on Women's Untapped Healthcare Needs are Transforming the Global Femtech Solutions". See: https://insights.frost.com/hubfs/Content%20Uploads/DGT/2021/HC/MFF7_Samples.pdf

3 "Digital Health Market Size, Share & Trends analysis Report By Technology". Forecasts, 2022–2030. See: https://www.grandviewresearch.com/industry-analysis/digital-health-market; see also: https://www.statista.com/statistics/1092869/global-digital-health-market-size-forecast/

4 Gambier-Ross, K., McLernon, D. J. & Morgan, H. M. "A mixed methods exploratory study of women's relationships with and uses of fertility tracking apps". *Digital Health*.

2018; 4: 205520761878507. See: https://doi.org/10.1177/2055207618785077

5 Savage, M. "The Swedish physicist revolutionising birth control". *BBC News*. 7 August 2017. See: https://www.bbc.co.uk/news/business-40629994

6 Lupton, D. "Quantified sex: a critical analysis of sexual and reproductive self-tracking using apps". *Culture, Health & Sexuality*. 2015; 17: 440–453.

7 Delano, M. "I tried tracking my period and it was even worse than I could have imagined". *Medium*. 23 February 2015. See: https://medium.com/@maggied/i-tried-tracking-my-period-and-it-was-even-worse-than-i-could-have-imagined-bb46f869f45

8 Tiffany, K. "Period-tracking apps are not for women." Vox. 16 November 2018. See: https://www.vox.com/the-goods/2018/11/13/18079458/menstrual-tracking-surveillance-glow-clue-apple-health

9 Kleinman, Z. "Femtech: right time, wrong term?". *BBC News*. 8 October 2019. See: https://www.bbc.com/news/technology-49880017

10 Goldhill, O. "FemTech is not and should not be a thing". *Quartz*. 3 April 2019. See: https://qz.com/1586815/why-femtech-is-a-sexist-category/

11 Tariyal, R. "To succeed in Silicon Valley, you still have to act like a man". *Washington Post*. 24 July 2018. See: https://www.washingtonpost.com/news/posteverything/wp/2018/07/24/to-succeed-in-silicon-valley-you-still-have-to-act-like-a-man/

12 Evans, D. "What if you could diagnose diseases with a tampon?". *MIT Technology Review*. 18 February 2019. See: https://www.technologyreview.com/2019/02/18/1326/what-if-you-could-diagnose-endometriosis-with-a-tampon/

13 Ibid.

Chapter 12

1 Dodson, Betty. *Sex for One: The Joy of Selfloving - Betty Dodson* (Three Rivers Press, 1987).

2 Herbenick, D., Fu, T.-C., Arter, J., Sanders, S. A. & Dodge, B.

"Women's Experiences With Genital Touching, Sexual Pleasure, and Orgasm: Results from a U.S. Probability Sample of Women Ages 18 to 95". *Journal of Sex Marital Therapy*. 2018; 44(2): 201–212. See: https://www.tandfonline.com/doi/full/10.1080/0092623X.2017.1346530

3 Green, P. "Betty Dodson, Women's Guru of Self-Pleasure, Dies at 91". *New York Times*. 3 November 2020. See: https://www.nytimes.com/2020/11/03/style/betty-dodson-dead.html

4 Russo, N. "The Still-Misunderstood Shape of the Clitoris". *The Atlantic*. 9 March 2017. See: https://www.theatlantic.com/health/archive/2017/03/3d-clitoris/518991/

5 O'Connell, H. E., Sanjeevan, K. V. & Hutson, J. M. "Anatomy of the Clitoris". *The Journal of Urology*. 2005; 175: 1189–1195. See: https://studylib.net/doc/8339689/anatomy-of-the-clitoris---journal-of-urology--the

6 Gould, Stephen Jay. "The Hottentot Venus." In *The Flamingo's Smile*, p.298 (New York: W. W. Norton, 1985).

7 O'Connell, H. E., Hutson, J. M., Anderson, C. R. & Plenter, R. J. "Anatomical Relationship Between Urethra and Clitoris". *Journal of Urology*. 1998; 159(6): 1892–1897. See: https://doi.org/10.1016/S0022-5347(01)63188-4

8 O'Connell, H. E. & DeLancey, J. O. "Clitoral anatomy in nulliparous, healthy, premenopausal volunteers using unenhanced magnetic resonance imaging". *Journal of Urology*. 2005; 173(6): 2060–2063. See: https://doi.org/10.1097/01.ju.0000158446.21396.c0

9 Wahlquist, C. "The sole function of the clitoris is female orgasm. Is that why it's ignored by medical science?". *Guardian*. 31 October 2020. See: https://www.theguardian.com/lifeandstyle/2020/nov/01/the-sole-function-of-the-clitoris-is-female-orgasm-is-that-why-its-ignored-by-medical-science

10 Hoag, N., Keast, J. R. & O'Connell, H. E. "The 'G-Spot' is Not a Structure Evident on Macroscopic Anatomic Dissection of the Vaginal Wall". *Journal of Sexual Medicine*. 2017; 14(2): e32. See: https://doi.org/10.1016/j.jsxm.2016.12.079

11 O'Connell, H. E. "Anatomy of the Clitoris". 2005. See: https://www.auajournals.org/article/S0022-5347(01)68572-0/abstract

12 Photograph: Marie Docher/Company Handout.

13 Sophia Wallace: CLITERACY. See: https://www.sophiawallace.art/cliteracy-100-natural-laws

14 Wahlquist, C. "The sole function of the clitoris . . .".

15 "Cliteracy". *Huffington Post* Projects. See: http://projects.huffingtonpost.com/projects/cliteracy/get-cliterate

16 George, C. "Meet The All-Female Tech Collective Taking Sex Toys into the VR Realm". *Sleek Magazine*. 28 March 2018. See: https://www.sleek-mag.com/article/motherlode/

17 Carpenter, V., Homewood, S., Overgaard, M. & Wuschitz, S. "From Sex Toys to Pleasure Objects". *Science Open*. 2018. See: http://dx.doi.org/10.14236/ewic/EVAC18.45

Chapter 13

1 "A Cyborg Manifesto: Science, Technology, and Socialist Feminism in the Late Twentieth Century." In *Simians, Cyborgs and Women: The Reinvention of Nature*, p.150 (New York; Routledge, 1991).

2 Clynes, Manfred E. and Kline, Nathan S. "Cyborgs and Space". *Astronautics*. 1960; 9: 74–76.

3 Cao, Yilin, Vacanti, J. P., Paige, K. T., Upton, J., & Vacanti, C. A. "Transplantation of Chondrocytes Utilizing a Polymer-Cell Construct to Produce Tissue-Engineered Cartilage in the Shape of a Human Ear". *Plastic and Reconstructive Surgery*. 1997; 100(2): 297–302.

4 Gnecco, J. S., et al. "Tissue engineered organoid co-culture model of the cycling human endometrium in a fully defined synthetic extracellular matrix". *bioRxiv*. 2021. See: https://www.biorxiv.org/content/10.1101/2021.09.30.462577v1

5 Wolff, E. F., et al. "Endometrial stem cell transplantation restores dopamine production in a Parkinson's disease model". *J. Cell. Mol. Med.* 2011; 15(4): 747–755. See: https://onlinelibrary.wiley.com/doi/10.1111/j.1582-4934.2010.01068.x

6 Santamaria, X., Massasa, E. E., Feng, Y., Wolff, E. & Taylor, H. S. "Derivation of Insulin Producing Cells from Human Endometrial Stromal Stem Cells and Use in the Treatment of Murine Diabetes". *Molecular Therapy*. 2011; 19(11): 2065–2071. See: https://doi.org /10.1038/mt.2011.173

7 "Who plays God in the 21st century?" *New York Times*. 11 October 1999. See: http://static.scribd.com/docs/7suj7h175bsf.pdf

8 Zhou, G., Jiang, H., Liu, Y., et al. "*In Vitro* Regeneration of Patient-specific Ear-shaped Cartilage and Its First Clinical Application for Auricular Reconstruction". *eBioMedicine*. 2018; 28: 287–302. See: https://doi.org/10.1016/j.ebiom.2018.01.011

Chapter 14

1 Reprodutopia: Design your future family. *NextNature*. See: https: //nextnature.net/projects/reprodutopia

2 Shulamith Firestone. *The Dialectic of Sex: The Case for Feminist Revolution* (William Morrow and Company, 1970).

3 Smajdor, Anna. "The Moral Imperative for Ectogenesis". *Cambridge Quarterly of Healthcare Ethics*. 2007; 16(3): 336–345. https://www.cambridge.org/core/journals/cambridge-quarterly -of-healthcare-ethics/article/abs/moral-imperative-for-ectogen- esis/B88576CE3AF545DF15E977212B709D5B.

4 Lewis, Sophie. *Full Surrogacy Now: Feminism Against Family* (Verso Books, 2019).

5 Dieke, A. C., Zhang, Y., Kissin, D. M., et al. "Disparities in Assisted Reproductive Technology Utilization by Race and Ethnicity, United States, 2014: A Commentary". *Journal of Women's Health*. 2017; 26(6): 605–608. See: https://www.liebert- pub.com/doi/abs/10.1089/jwh.2017.6467

6 Yu, L., Wei, Y., Duan, J., et al. "Blastocyst-like structures gener- ated from human pluripotent stem cells". *Nature*. 2021; 591: 620–626. See: https://doi.org/10.1038/s41586-021-03356-y

7 Liu, X., Tan, J. P., Schroder, J., et al. "Modelling human blastocysts by reprogramming fibroblasts into iBlastoids". *Nature*. 2021; 591: 627–632. See: https://doi.org/10.1038/s41586-021-03372-y

8 Aguilera-Castrejon, A., Oldak, B., Hanna, J. H., et al. "Ex utero mouse embryogenesis from pre-gastrulation to late organogenesis". *Nature*. 2021; 593: 119–124. See: https://doi.org/10.1038/s41586-021-03416-3.

Conclusion

1 Donna Haraway. *Staying with the Trouble: Making Kin in the Chthulucene* (Duke University Press, 2016).

2 Suzanne Anker. *Vanitas (in a Petri dish) 03*. 2013. See: http://suzanneanker.com/artwork/?wppa-album=20&wppa-photo=356&wppa-occur=1

3 Bigg, M. "IUD, You Owe Me". *Pulp Magazine*. 2020. See: https://www.thepulpmag.com/articles/iud-you-owe-me

4 Susan Squier. *Epigenetic Landscapes* (Duke University Press, 2017).

5 'Myconnect'. See: https://www.agapea.si/en/projects/myconnect

Acknowledgements

When we give thanks, we honour our origins and circumstance. Let me describe my own.

This book has many possible beginnings. One germ emerged during my PhD, which I would write from bookshops imagining the ideas I was nurturing would find a wider audience. And so I want to thank books, their writers, bookshops and the people who run them, for the hope and liberation they bring. I also want to thank my research group, the Reproductive Sociology Research Group at the University of Cambridge, in particular Professor Sarah Franklin, Dr Katie Dow and Dr Amarpreet Kaur for their scholarly guidance, moral support and friendship as I developed my ideas and grew my confidence during my degree and beyond.

Another possible beginning was the moment my agent, Eli Keren at London United Agents, recognised my little germ's lively potential and helped me find it a space to grow. In doing so he gave a story and its writer new life, and I will be forever grateful to him.

Once Eli had found my book a publisher, I had the pleasure of working with Hodder & Stoughton, and with my editor, Izzy Everington, in particular. Izzy guided me through the process with inspiring creativity, care and conviction, and I could not have wished for a better collaborator on this project – Izzy, thank you so much.

Then came the people I talked to as the book took shape. The activists, artists, researchers, and scientists, too many to name, whose thoughtful words and love fill every one of these chapters. They shared their experiences, their frustrations, but most of all their passion. As they spoke to me, I felt the force of the years of compassionate care they have all dedicated to the health of women, and the book was born in the spirit of that collective hope. I want to thank you all for the work you do, and for the time you have given me.

Then, I want to thank the women who have already engaged me in conversations about our health. As I began writing the story of our bodies, I began sharing my own experience in articles and conversations. In response, I received not only understanding but the generosity of others' stories in return. Through these exchanges, I began to see glimmers of the awesome, transformational power that connection through storytelling holds for women's health and quality of life. Thank you for writing this story with me.

Then, to circumstance. Mine has always been favourable, conducive to thinking and writing and making my way in the world. For that, I first of all have my mother to thank. Mum, thank you for taking care of me, for listening, for encouraging and sometimes even fighting for me. You have always encouraged me to be honest and brave, and with that you have given me everything I need. Dad, from across oceans, thank you for your love and support, and for believing in me more than I ever will in myself. My not-so-little brother, Bruce, your steady love and compassion have made this book, and these past years, possible – you're so much bigger than you know,

I'm so grateful for you. And to the rest of my family, from the gene pool and beyond – Carla, Marian, Auntie Janet, Bianca, Carmen and Izzy, thank you for your love and laughter that has given me a home wherever and however I have been.

My circumstances are, I know, entirely circumstantial. I have been so very privileged to have had the means and opportunity to think, write and live as I do. I want to honour that fertile soil most of all, and to cultivate it lovingly, skilfully, so that from it, more life can grow.

Index

Page numbers in *italic* refer to the illustrations